Handbook for Rediscovering Authentic Happiness in the Closing Years of our Life

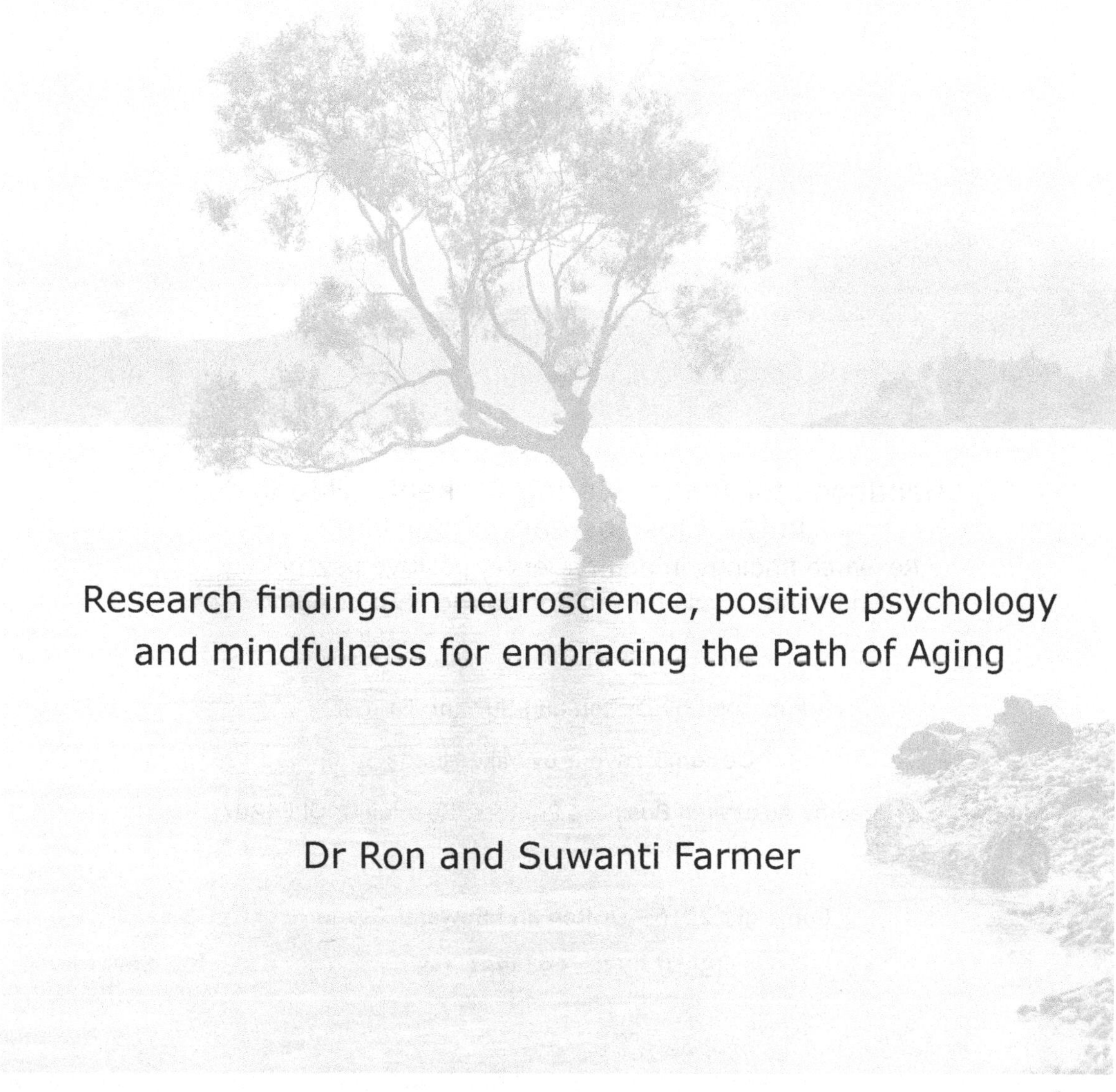

Research findings in neuroscience, positive psychology and mindfulness for embracing the Path of Aging

Dr Ron and Suwanti Farmer

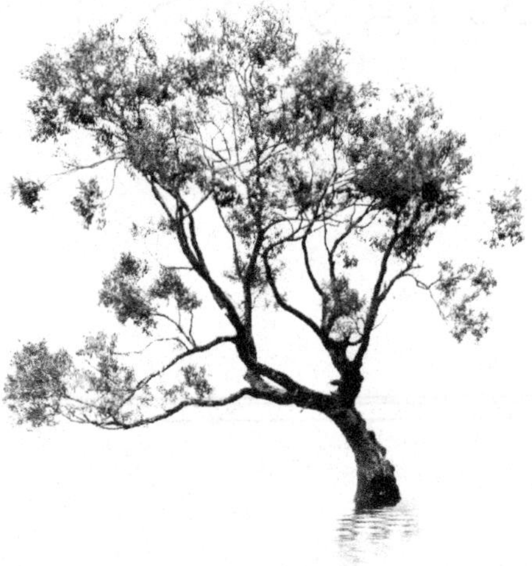

Handbook for Rediscovering Authentic Happiness
in the Closing Years of our Life
Research findings in neuroscience, positive psychology
and mindfulness for embracing the Path of Aging

Published by Dr Ron and Suwanti Farmer

Design & Layout by Mike Meade

Printed by Australian Business Printers, Beenleigh, Qld 4207

ISBN: 978-0-9944781-1-5

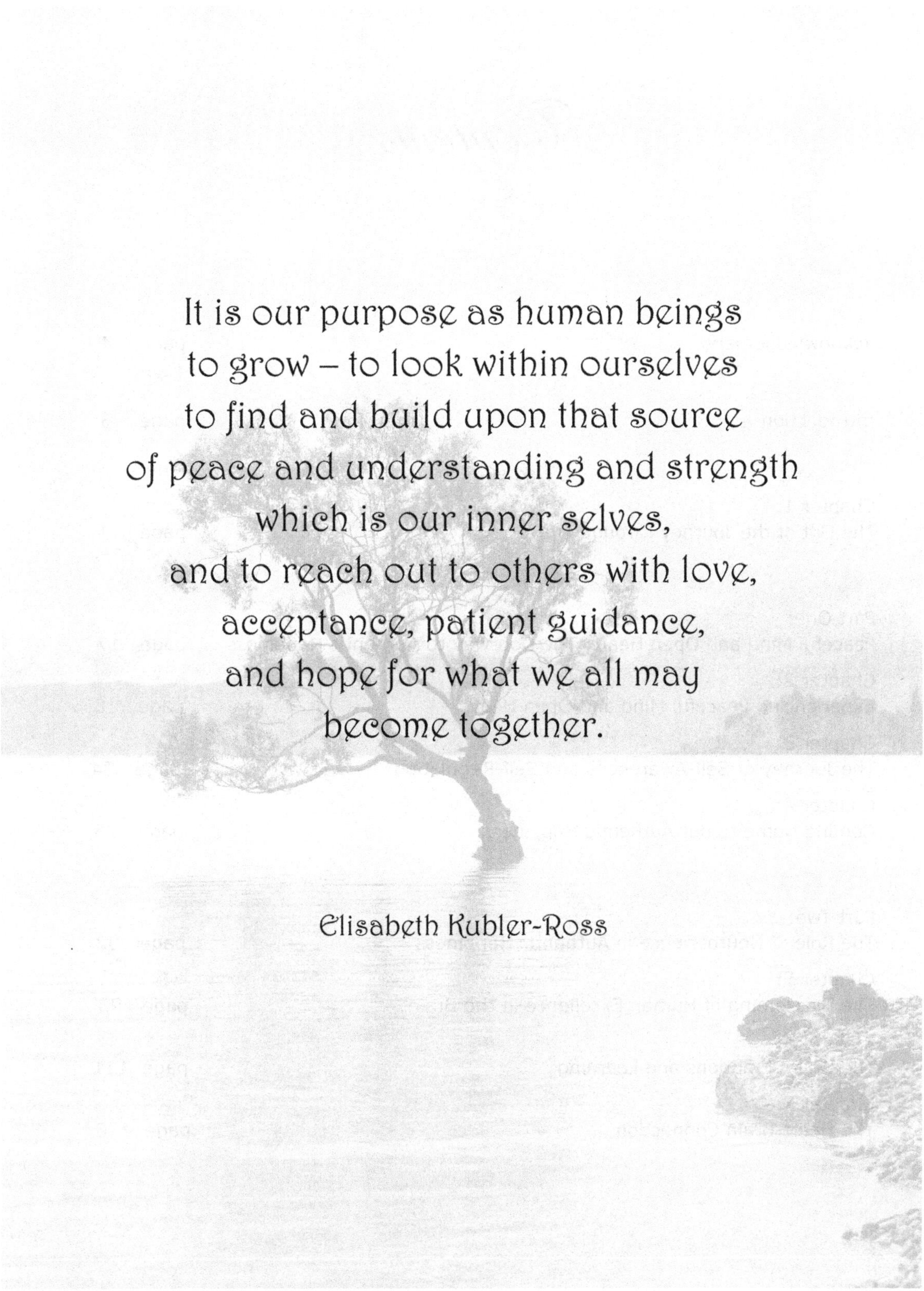

It is our purpose as human beings
to grow – to look within ourselves
to find and build upon that source
of peace and understanding and strength
which is our inner selves,
and to reach out to others with love,
acceptance, patient guidance,
and hope for what we all may
become together.

Elisabeth Kubler-Ross

Contents

Acknowledgements

Our gratitude goes out to SWAMI Home in Singapore – management and caregivers alike – for inviting us into their fold to learn and conduct training programs since January 2015. Without their example of meritorious aged care and collective commitment to self-transformation, this Handbook would not have come into existence.

We are humbly indebted to all of the writers and researchers in this important field whose work we have copiously drawn from; to Mike Meade for his tireless and selfless giving of time, energy and creativity in the preparation of the manuscript for printing; to Andrew Karydas and Sandra Taylor for valuable proof reading; and to our own parents and elderly friends who have shown us how to live, grow old, wane and pass on with such dignity, wisdom, humility and love.

Finally, we feel so blessed to have been given the opportunity to explore in depth the relevance of the five universal Human Values for personal renewal and for compassionate caring as explained so lucidly by Sathya Sai Baba, the international educationist and spiritual teacher.

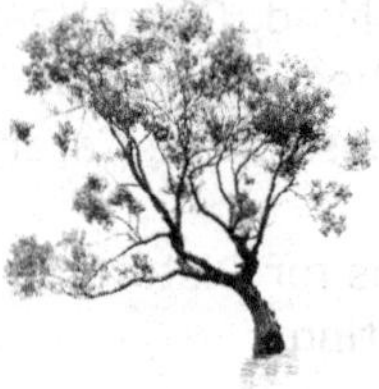

Introduction

May I be a guard for those who are protectorless,
A guide for those who journey on the road.
For those who wish to cross the water,
May I be a boat, a raft, a bridge.

Shantideva
The Way of the Bodhisattva

Along with his mentor Shantideva, who lived more than fifteen hundred years ago, the present Dalai Lama urges us to practise compassion, both for our own happiness and for that of others. The ancient wisdom consistently advises that pure love conquers all, in the same way that light always banishes the dark, without a struggle, and regardless of how black the darkness is.

When we banish all of the dark, only the light remains. When we bring love, peace, joy and gratitude into our life, this weakens and then banishes all of our fears, judgments and sadness, and every other cloud that hides the Sun of our supreme happiness, our inner peace, pure love and everlasting beauty.

We all want to be happy, and most of us want others to be happy. This is the quest that remains with us throughout every waking moment of our life. But how to do this? How to claim our throne so that we can wear the royal crown? How can we generate enough love and peace to expel what is weighing us down, those feelings and thoughts that keep us from flying to our Sun?

Essentially, this is what the present Handbook is about. It's to do with learning how to connect with that infinite source of happiness lying within us that is truly authentic, instead of with transient joys that are soon extinquished like candles in the wind.

That this is a lifelong journey of discovery, and not just a skill to be learned overnight, is made clear by the rising tide of depression, anxiety, addiction and suicide. Whatever it is that we need to know and learn, clearly so many of us are missing out on the Plan. It would seem that the more we are dependent upon the external for our happiness, the more we lose sight of the unbounded Treasure that is our birthright, a Peaceful Mind and Open Heart.

In many ways the material in the Handbook is to prepare us for the closing years of our life. What we learn now about 'The unchanging Self in the ever-changing flow of life' will serve us in good stead as we come into those years when the neurons in the brain begin to diminish and decay.

For all of us, the advancing years bring the news that the body, having reached its zenith in the second decade of our life, is steadily changing, leaving behind the form and function that might have been fashionable and agreeable to ourself. The now-commonplace resort to plastic surgery tells us how much we have colluded to reinforce this great fear of the unknown, the anxiety-laden question of, "What will happen to me as I grow old and then die?"

If our assessment of ourself is dependent upon the shape and function of the body, and what is acceptable in the eyes of the world, fear will arrive. Fear tells us that we are facing the wrong way; we have turned our back to our Sun; and, seeing the sad sight of our shadow, we spend our years running away from it. The great disappointment is that, however fast we run, our shadow stays right there with us, haunting us with its spectre of old age, dependency, loss of pride, weakness, and then demise.

If we think that we are the movie, there will be concern as it approaches the end. However, if we know that we are the ever-present screen upon whose surface these transient images of coming and going, joy and sorrow are being projected, there will be no room for concern.

The wise ones of old, like Buddha, Jesus, Krishna, Meister Eckhart and Guru Nanak, as well as those of more recent times, like Mahatma Gandhi, Eckhart Tolle, The Dalai Lama and Sathya Sai Baba, have all reminded us that we are the changeless Spirit, the eternal Witness observing all of our changes in thinking, feeling, doing and reacting. They have also said, in effect, that, 'What we are looking for, is what is looking.'

If we can remember to remember that within us is the Shangrila that we have been always seeking out there in the world, an awareness of lasting happiness will grow and ensue.

And if we can remember to 'wake up' to the Truth that we are the changeless Spirit, then the countless changes that come with each moment, minute, month and year will simply be noticed as they arrive, remain and then pass on by.

These principles are not always easy to accept and apply. However, we are blessed at this time in society's evolution that modern science is giving us new glasses, making it easier to see. Neuroscience, mindfulness, positive psychology and research into the aging process are providing us with fresh insights and techniques that bring ancient knowledge into a new light. This marriage of the old and the new forms the basis of what is offered in this present Handbook.

The world is a university, and life is a journey of discovery – one in which our mistakes are all opportunities to rediscover an authentic happiness that will continue to rise like the morning sun, even as we enter the closing years of our life.

My life when young was like a flower -
a flower that loosens a petal or two from her abundance
and never feels the loss when the spring breeze comes
to beg at her door.
Now at the end of youth my life is like a fruit,
having nothing to spare, and waiting to offer herself
completely with her full burden of sweetness.

Rabindranath Tagore

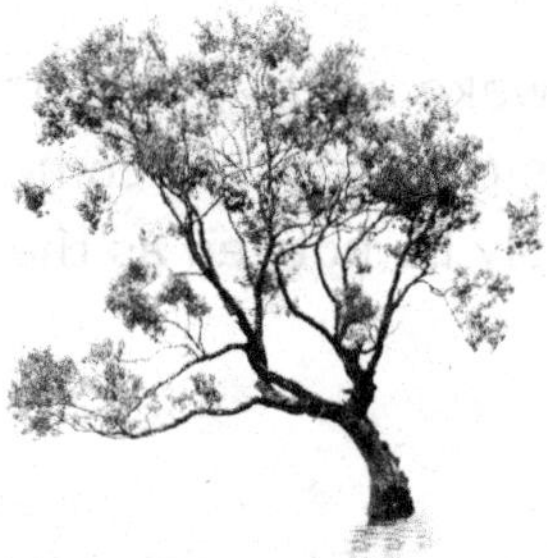

Chapter 1

The Gift of the Journey through Life

Thinking of myself as an ever-changing process
rather than as a fixed person
gives my life a feeling of fluidness and potential.
Toni Bernhard

It has often been said that Nature is the best teacher and also the best preacher. Reflecting on our human condition as we journey from birth to the closing years, we can look at any part of Nature and observe cycles of birth, growth and decay, and the decay is equally as important and beautiful as what came before.

Contemplating Nature, it is clear that the whole of life's journey – whether it be that of a butterfly, a tree or a mouse – is one of profound optimism and self-confidence. Consider a desert flower. It recognises that its beauty is unlikely to be noticed; it knows that its brief unfolding will be challenged by heat and then cold; and it realises that none will mourn its passing as it dries up into nothingness. Yet still it celebrates every step of its unique journey through life. At no stage does the desert flower doubt the reality of its own beauty and magnificence, even when only a skeleton of its once exquisite form remains. Oh, if only we could live like that simple desert flower, with such omnipotent self-confidence, such humility and optimism about the perfection of our own unique journey through life.

Some might say, "But desert flowers don't think." Certainly they don't think like we do, but 'think' they do, in ways that are incomprehensible to us, sufficient to survive under harsh conditions and to contribute in their own small way to the betterment of the whole, as does the most distant star and the least little blade of grass.

The powerful examples set for us by every part of Nature are legion, particularly in relation to healthy living, aging and dying. To take but one small but potentially life-changing illustration: no living thing - apart from humans and domesticated animals - eats more than it needs, and so we don't find obese lizards, overweight owls, tuna fish or goats. Why is it that humans disobey this common-sense guideline for healthy living? Perhaps it is because we seek a happiness that comes from without, one that is short-lived, giving way to disappointment as it loses its novelty or is no longer available.

In contrast, we know for ourselves that Nature is connected with its own inner contentment - one that never fades - which is why we yearn to be soothed and inspired by its Presence in gardens, forests, mountains and seaside retreats. Nature teaches by example. It prompts us to go within to find the Treasure awaiting us there. The poets have long said that the hum of the bees, the sound of the ocean, the croaking of frogs and the rustle of leaves in the wind are notes of the one divine melody that Nature is singing to us all. The refrain might well be:

Within you is pure, lasting, unsullied happiness.
Within you is a vast, limitless ocean of nectar divine.
Go seek it and find it, do find it.

If we could but follow this one example from Nature - that is, to be content with the 'what is', for that is the most holy - our sojourn through life would be satisfying and serene even during those darkest hours when we are compelled by fate to let go of all that we have delighted in, cherished and loved.

But how are we to turn away from what is so familiar, including our deepest fears and limitations, to embrace an elusive and unseen Treasure-house lying within while our bodies break down with illness or old age, our mental faculties decline, our control over life dissipates and the spectre of death moves ever-closer? How can we even begin to emulate Nature as it quietly celebrates the falling of its fruit to the ground where its perfect form disintegrates into a compost that nurtures new growth from a seed that has been hidden within? And how can we inspire and bring joy instead of grief to others with our passing, like the sun at the close of each day when it offers us its own requiem of countless, ever-changing patterns of indescribable colours, leaving us with a lingering yearning for what is Most High. If Nature is indeed our best teacher and preacher, surely there will be a way. And once we have learned to do this, others can follow behind.

Not too long ago we visited a friend's elderly mother who was dying of cancer in a hospital ward. Her children were concerned at the depth of her sadness and depression. She told us that she had nothing to live for, that every moment was nothing but a cruel imposition of fate. We said to her words to the effect of: "Your husband died when your five children were young and, by your example, you taught each one of them resilience, self-confidence, positivity and generosity. Now you have one more lesson to teach them before you leave this body." For the first time there was a spark of interest in her eyes as she turned to ask the question, "What could that be? How could I possibly teach them anything now?" We replied, with full conviction that she would rise to the occasion, "You have to show your children how to die." Within a week she left her hospital bed, involving herself in all of the joint families' activities, so full of joy and with an aura of unbroken serenity. She died three months later, having shown her children how to live life to the full in a body that was increasingly weak and dissipated, regarding death as the closing of one door and the opening of another. All she had been missing before was a sense of meaning: "Why am I here? What can I learn? What can I give to the world?"

After surviving years in a Nazi concentration camp Viktor Frankl (*Man's Search for Meaning*) wrote that those who had found a meaning for remaining alive were more likely to survive the starvation, typhoid, beatings and sheer horror of camp life. He asserted that we all have an inborn tendency to search for the light in a sea of darkness. However, when physical and mental privations accompany life's illnesses, aging and dying, it is not easy to remain focussed on finding the specks of gold that lie hidden amidst the slush in the bed of the stream.

There is a saying: "If you want to find a lasting contentment that remains with us every day, right through to our closing years, somehow we need to profit from the many thousands of little deaths that we are called upon to face throughout life." Every occasion of loneliness, betrayal, insult and injury, along with disappointment, pain, failure and loss, gives us an opportunity to undergo a metamorphosis, a crucifixion of the ego, compelling us to look within for what is being denied to us from without. We can share with you two powerful metaphors that illustrate this alchemical art of transmuting base metal into priceless silver and gold. One is called *The Sugarcane* and the other is *The Tree on a Mountain*. *The Sugarcane* one goes like this:

> Consider the plight of the sugarcane. Just when it is in its prime, growing strong and tall, someone puts a fire through it. Then it is hacked into pieces, crushed and then dried. So much suffering it has to endure. But in the end it triumphs, because what is left is sugar so sweet.

In the same way, it is the destiny of each one of us to undergo so many trials and tribulations throughout our life, as we age into our 70's, 80's and 90's . Our advancing years will at some stage see the burning of our hopes for a trouble-free life, the cutting down of our ability to achieve and excel, a crushing of pride in our looks and skills, and the drying up of our vitality, sense awareness, mental acuity and even perhaps our enthusiasm for life. If we can develop the conviction that our pains and sufferings come into our lives so that we can rediscover and identify with our 'sweet sugar' – our essential goodness, wisdom, love and beauty – then all of life's challenges will be seen as valuable, a gift of pain to break open our ego shell to reveal a treasure inside.

The second metaphor is *The Tree on a Mountain*. It goes like this:

> The tree on a mountain grows tall and can be seen from afar. The winds that blow at higher elevations are much stronger than the ones down on the plain, and it's for this reason that the trees on the mountain reach up so high into the sky. It might seem to us that the wind is the enemy of the tree, trying to uproot it from the ground. However, the tree regards the wind as its best friend. How could this be so? What really happens is that, each time there is another gust of wind, the tree bends to accommodate its friend and, in so doing, automatically sends its roots down deeper into the ground. There it finds more nutrients and water which it uses to expand its girth and grow even taller. The tree is so grateful to the wind for being the catalyst that triggers its rise to even more greatness.

The Tree on a Mountain metaphor is empowering for anyone suffering on many fronts – physical, emotional, mental, social and even spiritual – and for whom the onslaught of infirmities appears to serve no purpose other than to bring further despair and hopelessness. We might be caring for someone who is having their dignity and confidence stripped away by an ongoing deterioration in their health and wellbeing; or we ourselves could be assailed by sickness, a nervous breakdown, financial collapse, depression, work stress, stroke or a very uncomfortable aging.

Whatever the challenges might be, the sooner we can find meaning in each one of our afflictions, regardless of its intensity and duration, the closer we will come to our inland sea of undisturbed peace, and the more we will be prepared for an uncertain future.

There is a common wise saying: 'Always keep death over your left shoulder'. To our understanding, there are several levels of wisdom in these few words. The first is to remember always that the date and time for when we are to leave this body will always remain unknown to us, and that it could be tomorrow or even in the next hour. Reminding ourselves that we could have only a limited time remaining can act as an incentive to listen to our Soul's Compass, our Inner Voice, intuition or conscience which guides us in how to live an authentic life with a peaceful mind and open heart.

A second level of wisdom underlying the saying is that every moment is an opportunity for the ego-mind to 'die'. That is, every point in time provides us with a choice as to whether we shed another layer of our ego's skin: we can let go of an expectation, forgive someone, not judge that person, love more selflessly, avoid using hurtful words, enjoy a silent mind, show one more minute of patience, put off indulging this habit, let a desire fade, and so on through infinite possibilities.

A third understanding of 'keep death over your left shoulder' is to remember as often as possible that who we really are ('I', Spirit, Soul) does not die when the body dies, in the same way that when the movie in a theatre comes to an end the screen upon which it had been projected does not disappear. That is, to remember that we are not this body that thinks, moves and feels. Instead, we are the ever-present Witness who is observing this body's thoughts, feelings, actions and sense impressions. In later chapters we will return to this theme of the deathless Self, the unchanging Witness who is observing the changing scenes in this movie of life. This is an antidote for the poison of suffering; and it is a light that can give solace and meaning to those in the advancing twilight of degenerative aging.

The 'gift of the journey through life', the title of this chapter, is so often hidden from us. We are like the man standing at the door of his hut, hoping that some passer-by will offer a few crumbs to appease his hunger, completely forgetting that he had buried a priceless treasure just under the dirt floor. We are like the thirsty man standing waist-deep in a running stream of fresh water, oblivious to the gurgling abundance, holding out a cup for someone to give him some water to drink. We yearn for lasting happiness and unbroken peace, not realising that the purpose of our suffering is to turn our gaze inward to where our Treasure awaits.

The 11th century Sufi poet, Jalaluddin Rumi once said that "The thicker the lock, the more valuable the jewels that are secured behind the door." He also said, "The thicker the veil, the greater the beauty of the face hidden behind." There is such a measure of hope and optimism in these words. Our understanding of them is that our suffering is the 'lock' and it is the 'veil', signalling to us that something of great value lies waiting within us. Rumi's words also imply that the more intense and prolonged the suffering, the greater the inner riches and delights awaiting our discovery.

But how we are to gain access to this inner Treasure that is said to be our birthright? How are we to open the lock and lift the veil? Our beloved Rumi gives one more analogy to guide us in this endeavour. He says words to the effect of:

> When you find that your way to the Treasure is blocked by a heavy lock, or your gazing upon unsurpassed Beauty is barred by a thick veil, don't dwell upon the inconvenience of these guardians of the Temple. Focus instead on the priceless Treasure and the heavenly Beauty that lie beyond the lock and the veil. Then you will find that the lock and the veil are no longer obstacles, but instead benevolent signposts showing you the way Home.

If we can abide by the advice of Rumi and other wise ones throughout history who have left behind words of wisdom to guide us, we will discover that each step of life's journey is a gift, an opportunity to rediscover the essence of our universal, all-inclusive true Self: Peaceful Mind, Open Heart.

There is a light that shines beyond all things on Earth,
beyond us all, beyond the heavens,
beyond the highest, the very highest heavens.
This is the Light that shines in our heart.

Chandogya Upanishad

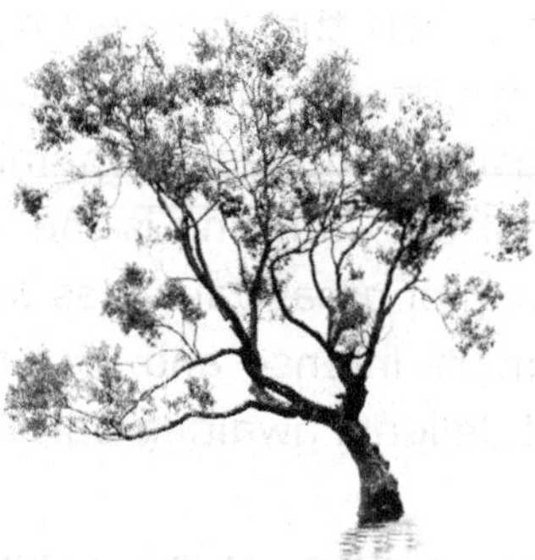

Part One

Peaceful Mind and Open Heart: The Doorway to Authentic Happiness

When the stories of our life
no longer bind us,
we discover within them
something greater.
We discover that within
the very limitations of form,
of our maleness and femaleness,
of our parenthood and our childhood ...
is the freedom and harmony
we have sought for so long.
Our individual life is an expression
of the whole mystery,
and in it we can rest in the center
of the movement, the center of all worlds.

Jack Kornfield

Chapter 2

Experiencing Peaceful Mind and Open Heart

Peace is present right here and now,
in ourselves and in everything we do and see.
Every breath we take, every step we take,
can be filled with peace, joy and serenity.

Thich Nhat Hanh

There is a 1200-year-old Shinto shrine outside Tokyo in Japan where the original cherry trees are as old as the ancient temple itself. The ragged decaying trunks still give birth to new shoots that grow into sturdy branches displaying clusters of cherry blossoms in the early days of spring. The gardeners lovingly fashion wooden crutches to support some near-horizontal branches, and they wrap hessian bags around the tree trunks to protect these 'old ones' from the harshness of winter.

These valiant survivors who were all once young and vibrant trees have made their annual offerings of exquisite flowers over many centuries. Each one can be seen as an artistic representation of how human aging can proceed. Although we might need increasing support and care as our body and mind decay, there is a beauty and dignity that can flower from within, again and again, seemingly without effort, for it is a spontaneous expression of our Essence, a smiling radiance from an ever-present, ageless spirit permeating every atom and cell of our living form.

It is the thesis of this Handbook – this approach to birth, life, aging and death – that as human beings we manifest our Essence, our inner Treasure, in varying degrees through the five universal Human Values of Love, Peace, Truth, Right Conduct and Non-violence which are umbrella terms for all of the noble human virtues lived at their highest levels. In our approach, we refer to the five Values collectively as Peaceful Mind, Open Heart.

It is our understanding that these Human Values can be identified as the pivot points of moral evolution, being universally accepted in their nature and manifestation. Recognised at the highest level in all societies and religions throughout recorded history, the five Human Values are the Golden Threads of the one Golden Cord running through the centre of what is good, best and most wise in all such groups of humanity.

Linking this observation with what saints and seers have asserted over the past few thousand years, we can say that, when the five Human Values are practised at the highest level, they describe a person who has discovered human excellence, one who is living a truly human existence.

Living a Truly Human Existence

Mystics have always said – and now scientists confirm – that every aspect of Nature has an inner blueprint that shapes its unique form and behaviour. A tree cannot grow into a bird and a fish cannot behave like a donkey. We are part of Nature too – in fact, as Henry Thoreau once wrote, we are Nature's way of looking at itself – and, in the same way that a mushroom, a platypus and an eagle behave truly according to their species, we can assume that there is a way of thinking, feeling, speaking and acting that is truly human. We are proposing that the five Human Values and the virtues subsumed under each one (e.g. compassion, humility, serenity, integrity, forgiveness, and so on) define such true human behaviour when neither ego nor attachments stand in the way of their full expression.

As we stand now, with all of our insecurities, impatience, judgements, desires and disappointments, we can imagine ourselves as a rough block of stone. In our preordained advance towards human excellence, we become the sculptors of our own personality, chipping away those thoughts, words and actions that keep us from identifying with our true Self – our Spirit, Soul or Essence – that can only manifest as Love, Peace, Truth, Right Conduct and Non-violence.

We are all destined to be engaged in this ongoing process of self-transformation. The grand cosmic design has given us agitation, sorrow, fear, grief and loneliness – in fact, all of the unpleasant emotions – so that we will be prompted to search for their opposite, in the same way that a fish out of water will struggle to return to the life-giving stream. Nobody wants to be unhappy and in pain, because we know with absolute certainty that our true nature is the antithesis of these disturbing states.

Our yearning to rediscover our true Self never really abates, although mostly we do not recognise that our pathos and discomfort is really the cry of the Soul calling us Home. We yearn to be loved, because we are Love – Love that is so pure and mighty that it knows neither boundaries nor limitations. We search for Peace, because our inherent nature is Peace – Peace that is so balanced and securely serene that neither trauma nor tragedy can disturb its constant equanimity - and so too for all of the Human Values.

We are drawn to hear, read about and be in the presence of those who exhibit advanced levels of human excellence, because we recognise our own potential in them. We see in them what we are yet to discover within ourselves. To the extent that they are manifesting Love, Peace, Truth, Right Conduct and Non-violence at a level that resonates with us, we yearn to experience such inner freedom and outer magnificence for ourselves.

Giants like Mother Teresa, Abraham Lincoln, Saint Francis of Assisi, Mahatma Gandhi, Albert Einstein, Florence Nightingale, Daniel Berrigan, Rachel Carson, The 14th Dalai Lama and Nelson Mandela provide examples of selfless service and compassionate leadership, those noble qualities that demonstrate the Human Values in action.

Such luminaries continue to be revered long after they have departed solely because they exemplified the art and science of being a true human being. They inspired a generation – perhaps several – to embrace a more elevated vision of humanity's inherent goodness and wisdom because they were all outstanding examples of the Human Values in action.

The qualities that enabled the Australian Aborigines to safeguard the environment of their vast land for 50,000 years are described by these five Human Values. The courage and compassion of those who laboured and fought to abolish slavery, overthrow Nazism, and develop modern social welfare lie within the realms of these Values as well.

If a garden is given sunshine, water and nutrients it will have healthy and vibrant plant life. Similarly, research is showing that those who cultivate Peaceful Mind and Open Heart are more likely to have enjoyable and fulfilling later years. To realise such a goal for ourselves, it is our understanding that the first step in this journey is to gain a deeper understanding of what each one of the five Human Values represents.

As will be seen in the descriptions that follow, each one of the five Human Values is regarded as having endless depth and breadth, like a limitless ocean – in the words of Ralph Waldo Emerson: "Under every deep, a lower deep opens" or, as the Sufis say, "When you peel a layer off an onion, you'll find there is yet another layer, then another, and another."

The Human Value of Love

ESOTERIC MEANING

In its esoteric sense, the highest Love is unbounded; neither increasing nor decreasing; constant as a fixed distant star. It is like the sun, shining equally on all, regardless of praise or censure. Love is nurturing, sustaining, attracting, expanding, unifying and self-sacrificing. Love is life. Who we are, is Love. All there is, is Love.

PRACTICAL MEANING

In practice, those seeking to live according to Love will try to be gentle, caring, empathic, compassionate and forgiving towards others. They will find joy in serving others; be loyal in friendship; practise tolerance and patience; and strive to restrain anger, greed, desire, envy and jealousy. They will be good listeners.

Looking for the innate goodness in all, and loving everyone the same, unconditionally, they will be happy for others' happiness. They will seek to overcome all difficulties with Love.

Love is patient, Love is kind.
It does not envy, it does not boast, it is not proud.
It is not rude, it is not self-seeking.
It is not easily angered, it keeps no record of wrongs.
Love does not delight in evil,
but rejoices with the truth.
It always protects, always trusts,
always hopes, always perseveres.
Love never fails.

Saint Paul's letter to the Corinthians

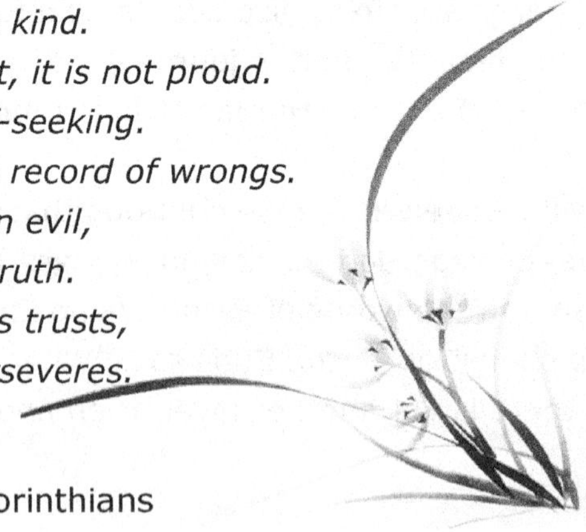

The Human Value of Truth

ESOTERIC MEANING

Scientists and seers remind us that we are all waves on the one vast limitless ocean of energy. It is this Oneness that defines Truth, often referred to as God or Universal Consciousness, the one Reality that manifests as all of this apparent diversity.

To know one's true Self is to know Truth, as when the bubble bursts it knows itself to be the entire ocean. We are not separate from anything or anybody; we are in every cell as life and in every atom as activity. I am in you and you are in me.

PRACTICAL MEANING

Those seeking to practise Truth will do their best to be honest with themselves and with others, and to be true to their word.

They will seek to develop their intuition, together with a sense of enquiry, open-mindedness, detachment and fearlessness; and will seek to discriminate between right and wrong by diligently listening to their conscience. They will cultivate the feeling of being connected to everything and everybody, remembering that what we do to others we are therefore doing to ourselves.

Truth is something that is not modified by
time or space or attributes. It must be
the same forever, unaffected and unchanged;
then alone is it Truth. It should not be
proved false by some subsequent
event or knowledge.

Sathya Sai Baba

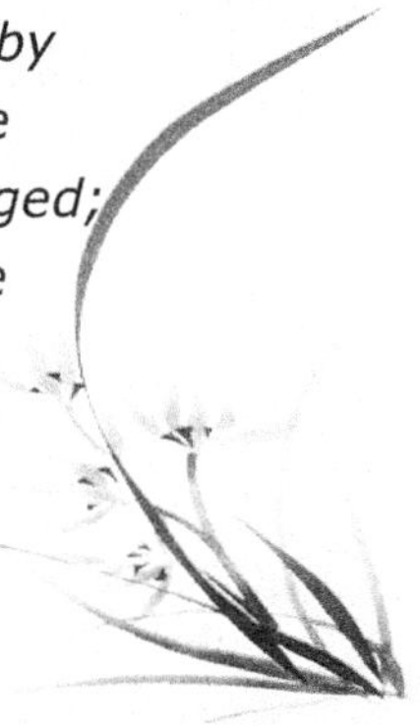

The Human Value of Peace

ESOTERIC MEANING

Abiding in perfect Peace, we are not troubled by fear, or desire, envy, hatred, greed or any of the tormenting passions – they are only transient mind-images on the unchanging screen of universal consciousness. We therefore experience unshaken equanimity, not swayed by praise or blame, profit or loss, joy or sorrow – regarding them merely as two sides of the same coin, for all is One.

PRACTICAL MEANING

In its practical application, those seeking to live in Peace will practise self-discipline, patience, tolerance and non-attachment.

They will think before speaking and acting; avoid or neutralise anger; place limits on satisfying their desires; learn to still themselves for reflection and prayer; try to love and serve all; and strive always to be true to their conscience. They will aim to regard all events as auspicious; develop humility; smile in times of difficulty; and cultivate optimism. They will remind themselves that Peace is to be found within and not outside oneself.

Great tranquillity of heart is his who cares
for neither praise nor blame.

Thomas a Kempis

The Human Value of Right Conduct

ESOTERIC MEANING

Right Conduct guides the whole universe – from atom to galaxy – in an exquisite dance of power and perfection. Every single thing is subject to rules that define 'correct action' in the context of its special place in the universe: its unique duty, nature and function. To align ourselves with the current of Right Conduct, we need to ask of each action whether it will lead us closer to, or away from, Love, Peace, Truth and Non-violence.

PRACTICAL MEANING

Those seeking to practise Right Conduct will show respect for society's laws, their parents and elders, and the customs and practices of other cultures and faiths.

They will aim to be healthy, hygienic, tidy, punctual, dutiful, reliable and responsible; to live simply; to study and work diligently; to respect elders; and to take on duties and responsibilities willingly. They will develop self-reliance, self-discipline and enthusiasm.

Underlying all this is a commitment to be true to the inner guidance of conscience, that which prompts all of Nature to be uniquely and perfectly Itself.

Your conscience knows the real source of joy; it will prod you towards the right path. Your business is to take it as a guide and not disobey it every time it contradicts your fancy.

Sathya Sai Baba

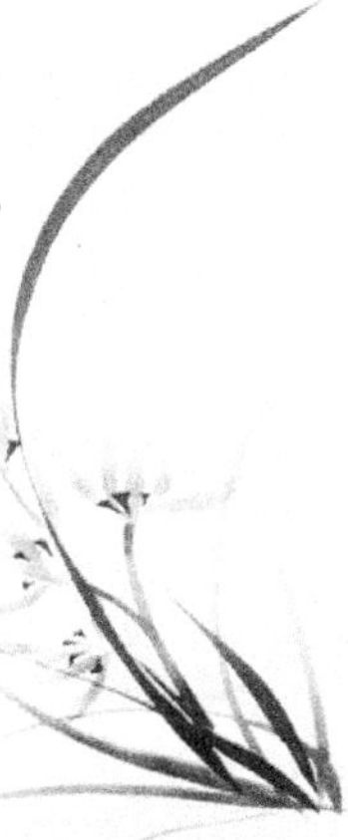

The Human Value of Non-violence

ESOTERIC MEANING

The two essential components of Non-violence are Understanding and Love. Understanding the Oneness of all creation nurtures care in our thoughts, words and deeds. The key to curbing violence is minimising ego-centred desires. Recognising our kinship with all of Nature, we hold to the supreme maxim: 'Help ever. Hurt never'.

PRACTICAL MEANING

Those seeking to practise Non-violence will try to avoid expressing anger, resentment, envy, jealousy and bitterness – instead, doing their best to cultivate Love and Peace.

They will cultivate gentleness, kindness and friendliness with all; having sympathy for the pain and difficulties of others – and so being unwilling to hurt or insult others in thought, word or action. They will avoid finding fault with others, and will practise forgiveness and forbearance when abused.

They will nurture loving concern for the natural environment, for all beings, all life.

An eye for an eye will only make
the whole world blind.

Mahatma Gandhi

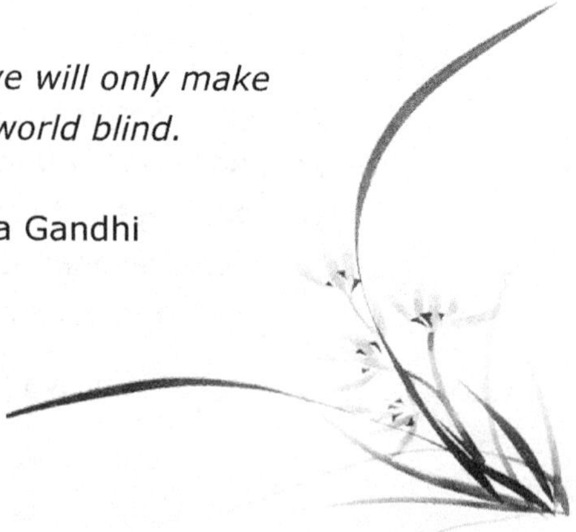

Each one of the five Human Values requires the other four Values to be present, otherwise it can only be regarded as diluted, contaminated by baser thoughts, words and deeds. In other words, we cannot assume that we are practising pure Love if we are being abusive to someone, dishonest, agitated or polluting the environment. Similarly, true Peace will not be present – even if we think we have perfect equanimity – if we are saying unkind things about another, inconveniencing others by being late, and so on.

To the extent that we are discovering finer and deeper levels of the Values within ourselves, in due course we will have Peaceful Mind, Open Heart – that state when all of the Human Values are being manifested in their full power and splendour.

Human Values are born with man.
They are not got from outside.
Man in his ignorance is not aware of these Values.
When man sheds his ignorance,
he will experience his divine nature.

Sathya Sai Baba

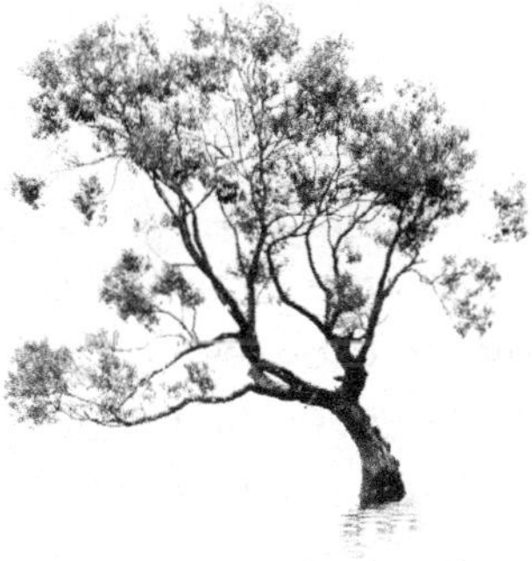

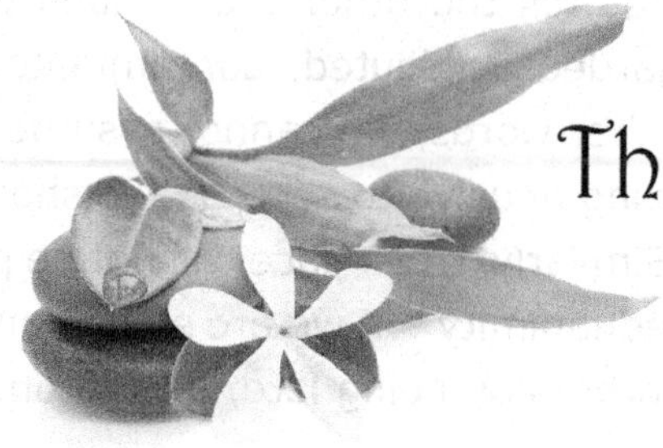

The Practice

EXERCISES FOR REDISCOVERING OUR INNATE HUMAN VALUES

Exercise 1:

Experiencing the Human Value of Love

Our long-term study and application of the five universal Human Values of Love, Peace, Truth, Right Conduct and Non-violence have led us to understand that they are a fine and workable description of the best that a human being can aspire towards.

The guided imagination that follows will open doorways in the mind so that we can catch a glimpse of the inner Treasure awaiting us all.

How can I do this exercise?

◇ Find a little time and a quiet place where you can sit comfortably as you read and imagine. Take your time with each step.

◇ Develop within yourself a feeling of pure, sweet Love. You might like to do this by recalling a time when you felt so full of Love.

◇ Allow this feeling of Love to grow as you imagine and experience some of the different aspects of Love. We'll start with Generosity.

◇ Imagine what it would feel like if you were really generous, always sharing – sharing your time, sharing your knowledge and skills, your possessions. What would that feel like to be so generous to those in need?

◇ Now add the virtue of Compassion.
Imagine that you have infinite compassion – for other people, for animals, for all of Nature.

◇ Now add the virtue of Self-sacrifice.
Imagine what it would feel like to be sacrificing your own comforts, your ego, and even your safety, for the sake of another person or other living things in need.

◇ Now add the virtue of Caring.
Imagine caring so much for the welfare of others that you can feel their pathos and pain, without being overwhelmed. Imagine caring about every single person on the planet, wishing them to have comfort and happiness.

◇ Imagine now loving everyone the same, as much as you love your dearest friend.

◇ Imagine feeling happy for people whenever you see them being happy, even strangers.

◇ Now imagine that every cell in your body, every thought, every feeling, is full of Love, full with all of these qualities of Love.

◇ Now imagine that this perfect Love is not only saturating your whole body, it is also above you and below you, expanding forever.

◇ Imagine that this pure Love is in front of you and behind you, stretching forever.

◇ And now imagine that this exquisite Love is also to the right and left of you, all the way to infinity.

◇ Imagine that you are immersed in a vast, limitless ocean of perfect Love.

◇ Say to yourself: "Love is within me. Love is all around me. I am this Love, everywhere."

◇ Come back to this moment, here and now, staying connected with the Love that you are.

Exercise 2:

Experiencing the Human Values of Peace, Truth, Right Conduct and Non-violence

This exercise requires quite a lot of writing, if and when you have the time.

How can I do this exercise?

- ◇ Study and reflect on the Human Value of Peace, as described earlier in this chapter.
- ◇ Using the style of the above script for Love, write your own instructions for a guided imagination of Peace.
- ◇ Take time to imagine as real, all of the instructions you have written on Peace.
- ◇ Now do the same, separately, for Truth, Right Conduct and Non-violence.
- ◇ Although this exercise will require quite a lot of time, the rewards will be great indeed.

Exercise 3:

Creating an Action Plan for each Human Value

Our wise inner Self is the one that knows the way Home. Through the self-rating approach in this exercise we will be guided as to what work we are ready to do on ourselves to live more fully according to our innate Human Values.

How can I do this exercise?

- ◇ Read through the table below (page 32) of the five Human Values and their Virtues.

◇ Decide on someone in your life whom you will focus on for this exercise. It could be a family member, a neighbour or any other person.
◇ Beginning with the Human Value of Love, give a rating for each one of the Virtues, according to how well you demonstrate that in your relationship with the person you have selected. The rating can be from 1 to 5, where 1 indicates a very low level of expression of the Virtue, and 5 indicates a level that any person would find welcome and admirable.
◇ Do the ratings for the Virtues that come under the umbrella of each one of the other four Human Values.
◇ For each Human Value, identify the Virtue that has the lowest rating. This will give you five Virtues to work with.
◇ For each one of the five lowest-rated Virtues, create an affirmation that you can repeat several times every day. For example, if 'Helpfulness' was the lowest-rated Virtue for Love, your affirmation might read: "From now on I will look for opportunities to be more helpful with (name of the person)."
◇ For each of the five affirmations, create an action plan to establish new habits for yourself, so as to ensure progress in expressing this Virtue. For example, if the focus for the exercise is on a work colleague, your action plan might read:
   1. Make it clear to Mary that I will always make time to help her with her more-difficult language studies.
   2. Act on any opportunity to help, whenever she is struggling.
   3. And so on.
◇ Having followed these steps for some weeks, you might like to extend them to the Virtue with the rating that is second-lowest, for each Human Value.
◇ If you find this exercise helpful, you could select a different person to focus on as you repeat the process; and then try someone else, and so on.

Just as treasures are uncovered from the earth,
so virtue appears from good deeds,
and wisdom appears from a pure and peaceful mind.
To walk safely through the maze of human life,
one needs the light of wisdom
and the guidance of virtue.

The Buddha

The Universal Human Values

Human Values	Virtues
Love	♥ Kindness ♥ Friendliness ♥ Caring ♥ Compassion ♥ Service ♥ Helpfulness ♥ Loyalty
Peace	♥ Patience ♥ Serenity ♥ Equanimity ♥ Humility ♥ Detachment ♥ Balance ♥ Forgiveness
Truth	♥ Honesty ♥ intuition ♥ Confidence ♥ Courage ♥ Idealism ♥ Trust ♥ Honour
Right Conduct	♥ Cleanliness ♥ Excellence ♥ Determination ♥ Generosity ♥ Integrity ♥ Trustworthiness ♥ Purposefulness
Non-violence	♥ Cooperation ♥ Gentleness ♥ Tolerance ♥ Respect ♥ Thankfulness ♥ Consideration ♥ Unity

Chapter 3

The Journey of Self-Awareness and Self-Regulation

The purpose of human life
is both personal and spiritual growth.
We are unable to grow toward greater understanding
of our true nature unless we take the time
to examine and reflect upon our life.
Examining our life reveals patterns of behaviour.
Deeper contemplation yields understanding
of the subconscious programming,
the powerful mental software that runs our life.
Unless we become aware of these patterns,
much of our life is unconscious repetition.

Robert Gerzon

To live with a peaceful mind and an open heart necessitates abiding in each one of the universal Human Values. Contravening or neglecting just one of the Values will agitate the mind and trouble the heart. For example, consider the virtue of honesty (an aspect of Truth). If we tell an untruth, our mind will always have to be on guard against exposing the deception, and our heart will close one of its doors so that we can distance ourselves from the other in fear.

You will see in Figure 1 that the first step in our progression towards uniting with the Human Values that lie within us (Peaceful Mind, Open Heart) is to focus on developing Self-Awareness. This provides the information required for Self-Regulation, which in turn gives us more opportunity to practise Self-Awareness – so it is a two-way process. Self-Regulation makes it possible for us to experience Peaceful Mind, Open Heart which is manifested in our lives as Authentic Happiness and Wellbeing, the Blossoming of Human Excellence.

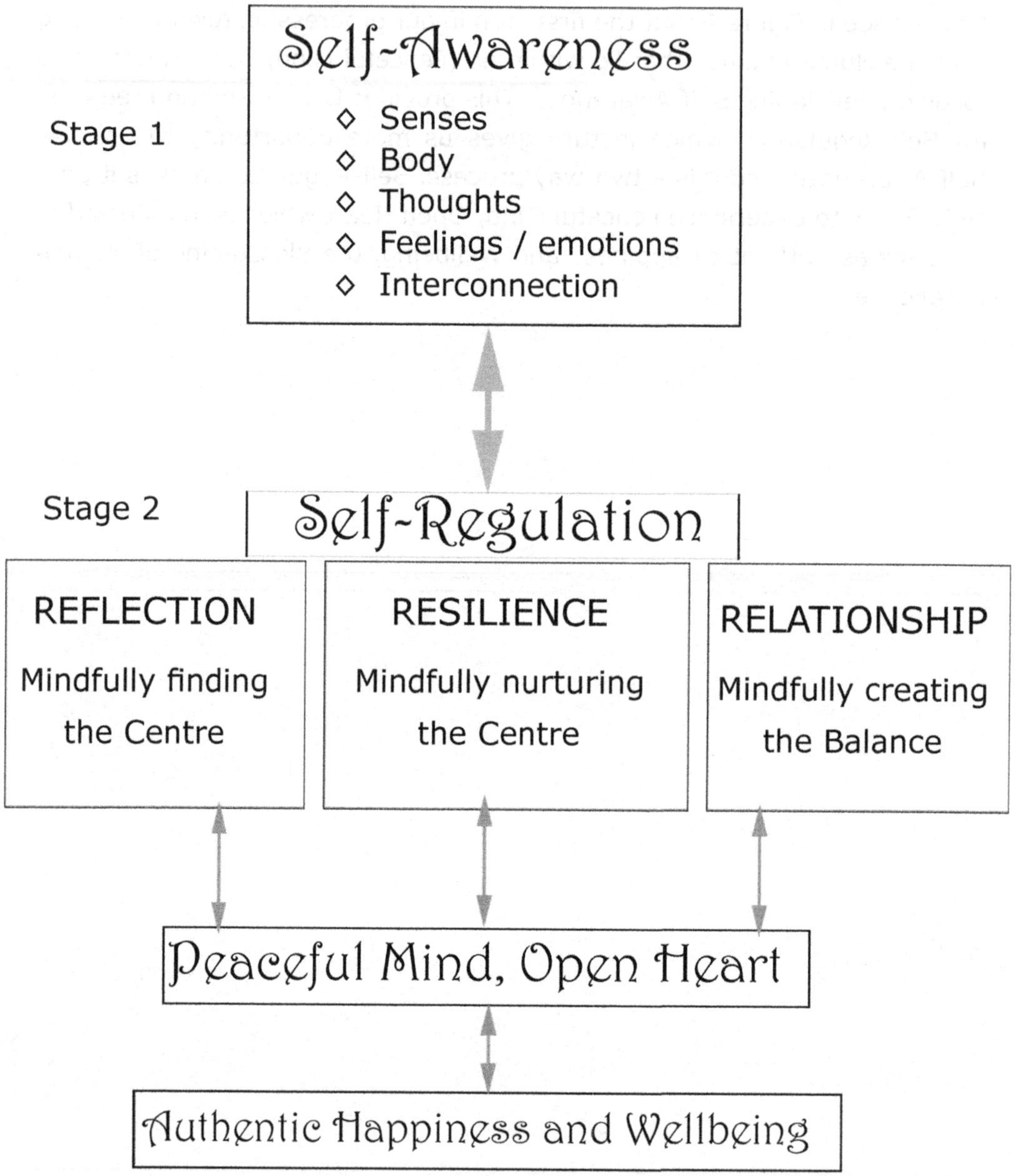

Figure 1: Model of Journey to Human Excellence through Peaceful Mind, Open Heart.

Self-Awareness

As the name implies, self-awareness is the ability to monitor our inner world, what we are experiencing, moment to moment. To a large extent, we live our lives only marginally aware of the information coming to us both interoceptively (inside the body) and exteroceptively (from outside). It is a form of 'waking sleep' - being awake but not aware of most of what is going on in our lives. Some of the foci for self-awareness are:

- ◇ Awareness of senses:
  what we see, hear, taste, touch and smell
- ◇ Awareness of body:
  what we sense in our bodily sensations
- ◇ Awareness of the experience of our thoughts
- ◇ Awareness of the experience of our emotions:
  naming each one, and noticing where it is felt in the body
- ◇ Awareness of our interconnections:
  our sense of relational connections with other people and Nature

Taking time to focus our attention in these different areas of our daily existence brings welcome feelings of safety and familiarity with our inner world, and provides opportunities for playing the game of life with more enjoyment and satisfaction. Casting the net of self-awareness a little wider, we move into the inner worlds of reflection and contemplation, looking at how we have been living our lives, wondering about our blind spots, waiting for insights to come that reveal some shadow that has been like a hand blocking our view of the sunrise.

The USA psychologist Martin Dresler has been applying neuroscientific methods at Donders Institute for Brain, Cognition and Behaviour to map out the functions of different parts of the human brain. In 2012, he and his colleagues identified a cortical network associated with self-awareness. It includes:

- ◇ Dorsolateral pre-frontal cortex:
  self-focussed meta-cognitive evaluation
- ◇ Dorsolateral pre-frontal and parietal lobus:
  memory demands
- ◇ Bilateral frontopolar areas:
  evaluation of one's own thoughts and feelings
- ◇ Precuneus:
  self-referential processing, such as first-person perspective
- ◇ Bilateral cuneus and occipitotemporal cortices:
  conscious awareness in visual perception

Decades of neuroscientific brain research tells us that neurons increase in number when a network is repeatedly activated, and decrease when it is left idle. So we can 'grow' our brain or let it decay, according to how much we exercise it. By engaging in self-awareness exercises, the neural pathways that govern this activity become increasingly more efficient – 'practice makes perfect' – thereby allowing us to become more consciously aware of our thoughts, feelings, bodily sensations, actions and connectivity, both within ourselves and with others.

In the mid-1990s, psychologist and science journalist, Daniel Goleman ranked self-awareness as the most important requirement for what he termed emotional intelligence – the ability to identify and manage our own emotions and the emotions of others – in the book of the same name. Neuropsychiatrist Daniel Siegel in his 2010 book, *Mindsight: The New Science of Personal Transformation*, links the practice of self-awareness – having insight into ourselves – with the ability to have a sense of the inner emotional world of someone else, thereby serving as a valuable tool for connecting with and understanding the person we are relating to.

Approaches for Developing Self-Awareness

◇ All of the mindfulness practices

There are as many ways of practising mindfulness – having the mind fully on the present moment – as there are activities that we can engage in, including watching the flow of our breath in and out of the body, noticing thoughts as they arrive and depart, and being aware of all of the sensations involved in eating, walking and so on.

◇ Journal writing

This involves looking within and reflecting upon events and how we reacted to them, as well as contemplating on unresolved issues, persistent thoughts and feelings. Writing about them in our journal brings insights and some detachment from disturbing feelings and memories.

◇ Self-monitoring

After selecting an aspect of our life that has a recurring, habitual quality to it (e.g. chastising someone, being critical towards oneself, and so on), we record on a spreadsheet each occasion of the event, noting the day, time, place and mental/emotional state at the time. This practice not only reduces the frequency of the habit, by defusing its unconscious power (like shining a light into a darkened room), it also increases self-awareness in other areas of our life as well.

Although practising mindfulness and other exercises in self-awareness offers rich rewards even by itself, progression from these to self-regulation brings us into the area of self-mastery – instead of being at the mercy of our thoughts, feelings, bodily sensations and what comes through our five senses, we move into assuming our rightful role of taking charge of those parts of our destiny that lie within our control.

Self-Regulation

To regulate aspects of the self – our habitual (often unconscious) patterns of thinking, sensing, feeling and acting – the essential prerequisite is self-awareness. Living according to the five universal Human Values is only possible if we have current information about how this human robot is already programmed. We are then in a position to change the program, to self-regulate, to change the course of the river of our life. As American writer and paediatric surgeon Bernie Siegel writes in his 1998 book, *Peace, Love and Healing*:

> *When we regulate anything, we need to monitor and then modify that which is being regulated. These are the two fundamental aspects of regulation. When we regulate our emotions, we monitor internal states and then modify our degrees of arousal and excitation to bring more balance into our lives. The outcome of healthy regulation is to co-ordinate and balance our functions so that we are adapting to our ever-changing environment in such a way that our innate Human Values come to the fore.*

In the earlier diagram we saw that self-regulation can be engaged in by focussing on one or more of three pathways:

REFLECTION	RESILIENCE	RELATIONSHIP
Mindfully Finding the Centre	Mindfully Nurturing the Centre	Mindfully Creating the Balance

Reflection, Resilience and Relationship are the three main pathways for manifesting our true nature, our Human Values, experienced as Peaceful Mind, Open Heart. Each pathway has its own importance and uniqueness. Consider this image as a way of illustrating each one of the three:

Imagine that the body/mind complex is like a pot of water in which we can see our reflection. The body is the pot, the water is our mind. When the water (mind) is still we can see our *Reflection*; we can see our beauty, goodness and magnificence (the five Human Values). This is *Finding the Centre.* There are so many pressures, temptations and old habits trying to lure us away from gazing within (into the pot of water), to experience our unchanging higher Self, our Human Values. *Nurturing the Centre* is how we engage in an inner struggle to stay connected with our Centre, to stay focussed within. *Resilience* has to be developed if we are to succeed in this endeavour.

For us to see our Reflection, the water must be still – any agitation distorts the surface of the mind and prevents us from looking within for our Treasure. So *Creating the Balance* is important, both within the body/mind complex, and between ourselves and others with whom we interact – that is, our *Relationship* with ourselves and with others requires balance.

Let us look into each one of these three aspects of self-regulation, these pathways to having Peaceful Mind, Open Heart.

REFLECTION : Mindfully Finding the Centre

Reflection is a way of attuning to one's own inner world such that social circuits of the brain are activated and developed. The result of teaching reflection as a basic skill would be the growth of the most human dimensions of our brains – our prefrontal cortex – while cultivating wellbeing in our minds, and kindness in our relationships with each other, and ourselves.

Daniel Siegel

Approaches for Mindfully Finding the Centre

Acceptance Commitment Techniques (ACT)

There is one particular set of techniques, well-researched by clinical psychologists, that has proved useful for *Finding the Centre*. The cluster of methods is referred to as Acceptance Commitment Techniques (ACT). Each one of the pratices leads to a deeper connection with our innate Human Values, our true Self that lies within us like red-hot embers hidden under the ash of a neglected fire. We can say that ACT removes the ash covering the fire. It dissolves the fears, agitations, avoidance patterns, negative attitudes and so on that have been keeping us away from our inner Treasure, our Human Values, our Peaceful Mind, Open Heart. We will explore ACT in a little detail.

ACT has six components. Application of even one of them can bring significant benefits. The six components are:

1. Defusion
2. Acceptance
3. Contact with the Present Moment
4. Values
5. Self-as-Observer
6. Committed Action.

We'll look at each one briefly, in turn.

Defusion

Neuroscientists have found that, when we engage in habitual types of thinking and reacting, the associated neurotransmitters in the brain become wired together (fusion) – 'Neurons that fire together, wire together' – making it more likely that we will react in that way again. Getting too close (attached) to our thoughts can be likened to touching a live electric wire and not being able to let go of it.

To rediscover our inner Peace and open our hearts to the Love that we are, requires defusion. That is, we can only look within to find these treasures if our thinking allows us to do so. Defusion lets us give less importance to our habitual thinking patterns, to distance ourselves from and to let go of unhelpful thoughts, beliefs and memories. In this way the neuronal pathways for those unwelcome guests are changed from a super highway to a seldom-trod bush track. To give three small examples of a defusion technique:

◇ Passengers on the Bus metaphor

This defusion technique helps us to ignore negative, self-destructive thoughts. The language used to explain it can go something like this:

> You are the driver of the bus and you know where you want to go. There could be some passengers on the bus who are calling out, "Don't go there! ... Stop here! ... Go faster! ... This is the wrong way!" Do you take any notice of them? No, of course not. Do the same with those thoughts that try to tell you to go the wrong way (e.g. "I might as well give up now. It's too hard," and so on). When such thoughts appear, just remind yourself, "They are just passengers on the bus. I am the driver and I know where to go, I am in charge."

◇ Shift and Shine technique

This defusion technique helps us to move or change a negative feeling to something positive (the meaning of the word 'shift').

First we shift the negative feeling and then, breathing through the heart, we think of someone or something that makes us feel happy. We feel that joyful feeling in our heart and then 'shine' it or send it towards someone or something special.

◇ The Leaves on a Stream exercise

For this exercise we imagine placing each thought that is noticed on a leaf and then watching it flow down a stream.

◇ STOP

We can practise the acronym:
Slow down and warm our heart (right hand on heart)
Take a deep breath through the heart
Open the heart to shine (spread arms out wide)
Picture a positive experience

Acceptance

We must not wish anything other than what happens
from moment to moment, all the while,
however, exercising ourselves in goodness.

St Catherine of Genoa

These words are in harmony with those of the mid-twentieth century mystic Alan Watts who brought esoteric Christianity, Zen and Buddhism to the youth of the West. He said,"The 'what is', is the most holy." It is a succinct way of saying that, as the Christian Scientists insist, only perfection exists, and that perfection is always present right now. This, as we see it, is the essence of Acceptance in ACT. Acceptance allows us to make room for painful feelings, urges and sensations – allowing them to come and go without a struggle.

If we have a feeling of sadness, for example, firstly we can observe it, accept it and make 'room' for it inside. We can see it as perfect from where we are right now. We can discover that the sadness is not who we are, but rather a doorway into the heart where we can feel a gentle compassion for all those who feel overwhelmed by an unbearable sadness.

Acceptance is a valuable self-help tool for anyone who is committed to living more fully the five Human Values – experiencing Peaceful Mind, Open Heart. It is a gift for all ages, giving them an appreciation of the 'What is' and the Now, the present moment.

Contact with the Present Moment

This component of ACT requires a certain vigilance to ensure that the mind's focus is on the present, not the past or the future. One of the most popular and effective means of doing this is the practice of mindfulness – of which there are many variations – whereby the attention is usually returned to a particular sensory or physical experience. We will be exploring mindfulness in some detail in later pages.

Contact with the Present Moment allows us to engage fully with the here-and-now experience, with an attitude of openness and curiosity. The ultimate purpose behind this approach is to find a more lasting and authentic happiness. As Lao Tzu, the 6th century BCE Chinese author of *Tao Te Ching,* advised:

> *If you are depressed, you are living in the past.*
> *If you are anxious, you are living in the future.*
> *If you are at peace, you are living in the present.*

When we endeavour to become proficient in 'being here for now' – as Baba Ram Dass, the former Harvard psychology professor, would say – the pressures of living are experienced in a different way, with less stress, more joy in the moment. Henry Thoreau wrote in Walden:

Above all, we cannot afford not to live in the present. He is blessed over all mortals who loses no moment of the passing life in remembering the past.

There are many ways of guiding us into the practice of mindfulness, each of which will give us the experience of being more in the present.

Values

If we can dare to live according to the values and virtues that resonate strongly within us, powerful things begin to happen. When we align ourselves with the current of our Soul's Compass it is as if all the forces of the universe rush in to support us.

The first step of course is to become aware of our own guiding moral principles. If one of them is kindness, we can ask: "Am I being equally kind to all, particularly those who have been unkind to me?"

It requires conviction and courage to commit ourselves to living the values we believe in, wherever that path may take us. If we can do this, what we share with others will have far-reaching effects upon their future and that of society. Henry Thoreau said it well:

If a man loses pace with his companions, perhaps it is because he hears a different drummer. Let him step to the music he hears, however measured, or far away.

Self-as-Observer

There is an encouraging trend in a few sectors of psychology, education and mental health where researchers have cast their nets wider to embrace some of the central tenets of Eastern spirituality. Mindfulness has been their most visible adoption, arriving like an incoming tide to lift the discourse and techniques applied in these fields. Lesser known has been the advent of Self-as-Observer. Eighty years ago, Ramana Maharshi said:

> *You have to ask yourself the question, "Who am I?" This investigation will lead in the end to the discovery of something within you which is behind the mind. Solve that great problem, and you will solve all other problems thereby. Man's real nature is happiness. Happiness is inborn in the Self. His search for happiness is an unconscious search for his true Self. The true Self is imperishable; therefore, when a man finds it, he finds happiness which does not come to an end.*

Practice of Self-as-Observer allows us to experience a sense of Self, from which to observe and accept all changing experience. It allows us to relate to that same Self in others, ignoring the negativity, seeing only the goodness, relating to their wise inner Self; and knowing that – as for ourselves – who they really are is not affected in any way by their suffering or despair.

The ideal analogy for Self-as-Observer is the movie screen which is not affected by the fire and floods depicted in the movie. The screen is not burned, nor does it get wet, and, like the true Self, is no longer visible once the movie (of life) has started. In the same way, the higher Self, largely hidden from our everyday self, remains ever-serene and content, unaffected by the ups and downs of life. We are the screen, not the movie; we are the Self-as-Observer, not that which we are observing (our thoughts, feelings, etc.).

Committed Action

One aspect of the Human Value of Right Conduct says:

> When we know what action needs to be taken,
> begin as soon as possible.

When we know what activity we should not be engaging in,
cease doing it immediately.
When we are not sure what to do, wait.

The Wise One within knows the Path that has to be followed to find our Centre, our Peaceful Mind, Open Heart. Too often we neither listen to nor obey these dictates of the Soul's Compass, even going against the values we have resolved to live by. Lack of any lasting and authentic happiness is the end result of such wilful negation – it is as if we turn our back to our Sun, preferring instead to stay with the familiarity of our 'shadow', those life-long fears and indulgences that follow us through life like a burdensome companion.

In contrast, when we do engage in Committed Action, choosing to face our Sun and live according to our higher values, we reap the untold benefits that come to those who dare to leave behind the comforts of the 'known' as they step out onto the Path that leads to their Centre, the vast unknown of the true Self – Peaceful Mind, Open Heart.

To the extent that we can live by Committed Action, the unspoken message of righteous living given to others by our example will open doors in their minds and hearts, allowing them to connect with their own deeper levels of nobility, courage and determination to commit themselves to act on their chosen values.

Let us rid ourselves
of all things that hinder us
and run with courage and endurance
the race that is set before us.

Hebrews 12:1

Nurturing the Centre (Resilience) can be likened to building a boat to sail across the ocean of life. Without the boat, we are struggling in the water, with waves (of emotion) threatening to engulf us, and sharks (self-defeating thoughts) attacking us at any time. So long as we are 'sitting in our boat' (in our safe, calm, inner Centre) the presence of unsettling emotions (the waves) and disturbing thoughts (the sharks) will not affect us. Regardless of the challenges facing us, we are safe if we can sit in our boat, regulating how we think, feel and behave.

Approaches to Mindfully Nurturing the Centre

There are a number of useful pathways we can follow to ensure that we can remain in – or return to – our Centre. Each one is a form of resilience.

(A) The Five C's of Resilient Coping

Based on the latest findings of neuroscience, Linda Graham in her 2013 book, *Bouncing Back: Rewiring Your Brain for Maximum Resilience and Wellbeing,* outlined the five C's of resilient coping. Each one of these can be recognised as a sub-value of one of the five Human Values. The five C's are:

1. Calm (Peace)
   To stay calm in a crisis

How to do this?

o Mindfulness of breathing

Regular practice of mindful-breathing exercises during the day gives us the growing conviction that there is a Calm centre within us that can be connected with at any time, most of the time, particularly during those challenging periods when we find ourselves yet again in the 'water' struggling to return to the safety of our 'boat' – where Peaceful Mind, Open Heart reigns supreme.

o Body scan

This technique involves 'paying attention on purpose' for a few seconds to a sequence of body parts (e.g. "Bring your attention to your right foot ... your right ankle ... your right calf muscle ..." and so on), without trying to relax them.

It takes us underneath the incessant waves of thinking on the surface of our mind into that space of inner silence and tranquillity. Becoming familiar with this inner world of stillness and serenity is an important ingredient in the rich mix of resilience.

2. Clarity (Truth)

To see clearly what's happening as well as to be aware of our internal response to what we are witnessing; to see what needs to happen next; and to look at the situation from different perspectives so that we can enhance our ability to respond in a flexible way

How to do this?

o Cultivating equanimity

Our challenge is to learn how to develop and remain in a state of equanimity, so that we cannot be swayed by any tricks of the mind trying to catastrophize a present or a possible future.

Certainly, frequent practice in mindfulness gives the nervous system the reassurance that 'fight or flight' is not necessary. However, the habitual thought patterns also need to be modified or reduced, to be replaced by an ongoing attitude such as 'everything has its opposite', 'there are always two sides to the story', 'after the tide goes out, it always comes in again', and so on.

o Resonating with the calm of others to calm ourselves down
When we get distressed, worried, disappointed, fearful or confused, we can see all of these as opportunities for us to learn resilience – to stay steady on the course without being swayed by external events or self-doubt issues. One way to do this is to imagine being in the presence of an admired figure who is always steady, radiating equanimity and resilience, regardless of the storms and tempests of life pounding away at them.

3. Connection (Love)
To reach out for help as needed; to learn from others how to be resilient; to connect to resources that greatly expand our options

How to do this?

o Nurturing gratitude
It is not generally recognised that the Human Value of Love has great power. When our heart is open in Love towards ourselves, others and the universe, trust is present and fear is absent. Simply by listing thirty things we can be grateful for (e.g. I am alive, I heard a bird sing, someone smiled at me, I have food to eat, and so on), and another thirty kind things that others have done for us (e.g. someone held open a door for me; my brother wrote to me; and so on), already our heart has opened enough to counteract any thoughts of gloom and doom.

o Creating material resources
Each of us can use our creative and investigative skills to identify

activities and materials that promote and teach about resilience (e.g. Google: 'Ten ways to build resilience').

- Discovering people as resources
  Although it might take a little time to do this, we have those people in our lives who are like-minded and committed to living a values-focussed life. Amongst them will be some to whom we can go when we are in need of support, advice or reassurance, when we feel like there is an impasse, confusion or catastrophe that is challenging our self-confidence or our will to push on and to keep going.

4. Competence (Right Conduct)
   To call on skills and competencies that have been learned through previous experience that allow us to act quickly and effectively

How to do this?

- Identify earlier examples of resilience
  When events conspire to overwhelm us so that we feel defeated and down, unable to cope, it is important to cast our mind back through our life to an earlier time when a tidal wave of misfortune descended upon us. Somehow we survived and perhaps even gained something of value. What did we do then? Did we pray, get physically fit, go away for a few days, talk to a friend? There will be something that reveals itself, an aspect of resilience that gave us the courage and strength to persevere, be positive, or discover an inner faith and trust in a benevolent universe. Once identified, we can build on that skill, that wisdom, to face our present circumstances.

- Honouring the innate goodness of others
  This recognition of Truth – that a 'diamond' lies (sometimes hidden) within each and every person – releases the constraints on the flow

of energy and strength that is required to persevere against the buffeting winds of self-doubt and the powerful tides of the opinions of others. Affirming that everyone is doing the best that they can to be good, kind and loving – even the most cruel murderer, who is plagued by ignorance and fear – removes the impediments and weakness of will that come with failing to see the perfection in all beings, all events.

5. Courage (Non-violence)
   To strengthen the faith to persevere in the actions until we come to a resolution or acceptance of the difficulty

How to do this?

- I am ready for this
  In the same way that students are only examined upon the material they have been learning throughout the year, the challenges presented to us are what we are ready for. That is, given all of the wisdom and skills that we have learned to date, whatever life presents to us is what we are ready for. Such an attitude is very empowering. Having the conviction that this challenging situation is but an opportunity to put into practice what we already know banishes feelings of self-doubt, self-pity, anxiety and being overwhelmed. By silently affirming, "I am ready for this," and even, "Thank you for this test," we open our mind and heart to the untapped power and strength lying within us.

(B) Bounce Back Program

A well-tested, self-help program for developing resilience was devised by two Australian psychologists, Helen McGrath and Toni Noble. The syllables in the words BOUNCE BACK form the acronym for the ten mental attitudes that have been shown to enhance resilience. They are:

Bad times don't last. The tide always turns and comes in again.

Other people can help if we share our concerns with them.

Unhelpful thinking makes us even more upset.

Nobody is perfect in these human forms.

Concentrate on positive thinking.

Everybody has disturbing thoughts and feelings at times. They always pass.

Blame fairly – How much of what happened was because of ourselves, others or fate?

Accept the things we can't change, while changing those we can.

Catastrophizing exaggerates our difficulties. We do not have to believe the worst story in our head.

Keeping things in perspective. This is just one part of my life. I will not let it spoil the rest.

(C) Healthy Mind Platter

Another strategy for developing resilience is the Healthy Mind Platter presented by two neuroscience experts, David Rock and Daniel Siegel. The seven practices all strengthen those parts of the brain that create resilience. They are:

Focus Time:
When we focus closely on tasks in a goal-oriented way, we take on challenges that make deep connections in the brain.

Play Time:
When we allow ourselves to be spontaneous or creative, playfully enjoying novel experiences, we help make new connections in the brain.

Connecting Time:
When we connect with other people (ideally in person), and when we take time to appreciate our connection to the natural world around us, we activate and reinforce the brain's relational circuitry.

Physical Time:
When we move our bodies, aerobically if medically possible, we strengthen the brain in many ways.

Time In:
When we quietly reflect internally, focussing on sensations, images, feelings and thoughts, we help to better integrate the many different components in the brain.

Down Time:
When we are non-focussed, without any specific goal, and let our mind wander or simply relax, we help the brain recharge.

Sleep Time:
When we give the brain the rest it needs, we consolidate learning and recover from the experiences of the day.

We all know from our own experience that each one of these, if neglected, can result in a diminution in resilience, a reluctance to keep going and persevere.

RELATIONSHIP: Mindfully Creating the Balance

This is the third of the inter-related components for activating Self-Regulation.

> *Relationship experiences have a dominant influence on the brain because the circuits responsible for social perception are the same as or tightly linked to those that integrate the important functions controlling the creation of meaning, the regulation of bodily states, the modulation of emotion, the organization of memory and the capacity for interpersonal communication. Interpersonal experience plays a special organizing role in determining the development of brain structure early in life and the ongoing emergence of brain function throughout the lifespan.*
>
> Daniel Siegel

Our brain has many different parts with different responsibilities. The key to thriving is to help these parts work well together – to integrate them, for them to have a good relationship with each other. Integration takes the distinct parts of our brain and helps them work together as a whole. Integration is simply that: linking different elements together to make a well-functioning whole. Integration coordinates and balances the separate regions of the brain that link together.

It is possible for our brain to become more integrated and for us to use our mental resources to a greater capacity - this increases the quality of our lives. Simply by being present in the Now, in the present moment, within our interactions with others, the different parts of our brain become better integrated. As a result, because of the improved quality of our relationships, we will thrive emotionally, intellectually, and socially. Having an integrated brain allows us to have improved decision making, better control of the body and emotions, fuller self-understanding, stronger relationships, and success in life.

When we react to a situation and get stuck in distress, worry, upset, anger, frustration or trauma, our brain, mind and body are dis-integrated. There is a thought, or feeling, or memory that has hijacked us and is running the show, preventing us from thinking clearly or behaving appropriately. To reintegrate requires an understanding of what is happening so that we can make a choice to use tools that can help 'shift' the brain physiology – allowing the body to calm, the heart to open, and the right, left, lower, middle, and upper parts of the brain to reconnect.

Approaches for Mindfully Creating the Balance

(A) Techniques for harmonious integration

A number of relationship-based strategies for reintegrating those parts of the body and brain that return balance to the nervous system have been developed by different researchers. Daniel Siegel and Tina Bryson have outlined in their 2011 book, *The Whole Brain Child*, a number of strategies for re-establishing harmonious integration in the brain. Some of these are :

1. Connect and redirect
2. Name it to tame it
3. Engage the upstairs brain
4. Move the body
5. Acts of compassion and forgiveness

1. Connect and redirect
   Example of activity: instead of command and demand, try to connect and redirect

   The essence of this approach is that responding with logic (left brain) to others when they are angry, anxious or withdrawn will often not work until we have addressed the right brain's emotional needs. That is, we need to connect first with the person through empathic listening and understanding. This brings the two sides of the brain into balance so that now reason and logic (left brain) can be brought in to redirect the person's focus onto possible solutions for their concerns.

2. Name it to tame it
   Example of activity: instead of dismiss and deny, try name it to tame it

   Because it is the right hemisphere in the brain that forms a feedback loop with the amygdala (the 'seat of emotion') so as to ensure that a frightening or painful experience can be avoided in the future, it does not have the ability to apply the brakes to this function. It is the left hemisphere's role to do this. Our strategy here is to encourage the person to retell the story of the misfortune (with some assistance) again and again until the left brain activity has balanced that of the right, allowing feelings of peace and safety to return. Alternatively, the person can be encouraged to draw a picture of the trauma, or write about it. Talking, drawing or writing about what happened is like giving a name to the distressing emotions (the left brain is highly literate) and in this way they are tamed, no longer dominating.

3. Engage the upstairs brain
   The nine functions of the pre-frontal cortex (Upstairs Brain)

   Although every part of the brain plays its own important role in the energising and regulating of the whole mind/body/relationship complex, it is the pre-frontal cortex that plays the most critical role in the development of our character traits, such as the degree to which we can live according to our Human Values. This middle pre-frontal region of the brain is where life-changing decisions are made and ethical/moral behaviour is mediated.

The cluster of neurons included in the pre-frontal cortex have at least nine important functions, each of which are involved in our quest to develop the best possible relationships with others. We will explore these functions in more detail in Part Two in this Handbook.

It is known that both empathy and mindfulness help develop all nine functions of the pre-frontal cortex, which in turn create and strengthen new pathways for ensuring effective relationships with others. By giving attention to each one of those nine functions, we will be strengthening the same pathways of the brain that will assist us to become aware of what we are experiencing, an invaluable gift for any human being.

4. Move the body

Nearly fifty years ago researchers in psychosomatic medicine discovered that, for every thought and emotion that we experience, there is a specific pattern of minute muscular contractions that work to maintain that attitude or feeling, different for each individual. The implication of these findings is that, if we can interfere with the set muscular pattern that supports the disturbing thought or emotion – by engaging in vigorous exercise for a few minutes – this makes it easier for us to move out of that locked-in state.

When there are strong negative thoughts, feelings, words and actions disturbing the harmony of our relationships with others, we can use this knowledge to help us move towards having a more Peaceful Mind and Open Heart.

5. Acts of compassion and forgiveness

Compassion and forgiveness both trigger the heart to send special signals to the brain so that it can help us to let go of a habitual negative reaction to something happening in our relationship with another person. The old adage of 'put yourself into the shoes of another' changes our perspective so that we can imagine, feel and see the suffering that the other person might be experiencing. This softens our heart still further until we can see once again that love and harmony are the only real feelings that matter.

Another familiar wise saying repeats the words of Jesus as he was being crucified: "Forgive them for they know not what they do." Allied to this is the reminder that 'The blind man cannot see. Even if he wants to see, he remains blind.' These understandings usher in forgiveness, that healing balm for those 'wounds' of ours that still cause us emotional pain.

(B) Five keys for harmonious relationship

So much discord and misery in the world comes about through lack of harmony in our relationships with others. If we can learn the art of self-regulation in how we interact with our families, friends and strangers we will have taken giant steps towards rediscovering our inborn Peaceful Mind, Open Heart.

In his 2002 book, *How to Be an Adult in Relationships*, psychologist David Richo identified five keys or prerequisites for a mindful, harmonious and richly-rewarding relationship with others. They are:

- Attention to the present moment
- Acceptance of self and others

dices, so that we can be open to the unfolding of possibilities of the present moment

Each of the five keys opens a doorway into another level of good-quality relationships. We can reflect on how each one can be applied in particular relationships, either in real life or imagination. It requires us to be mindful, carrying out internal searches to see how we are going. We will return to these five keys for a mindful relationship in The Practice section to follow.

This above all:
To thine own self be true.
And it must follow,
as the night the day,
thou canst not be false to any man.

William Shakespeare

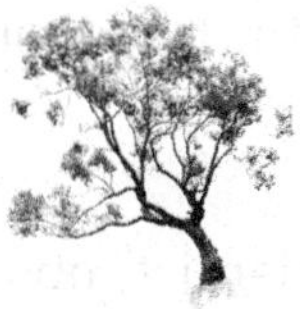

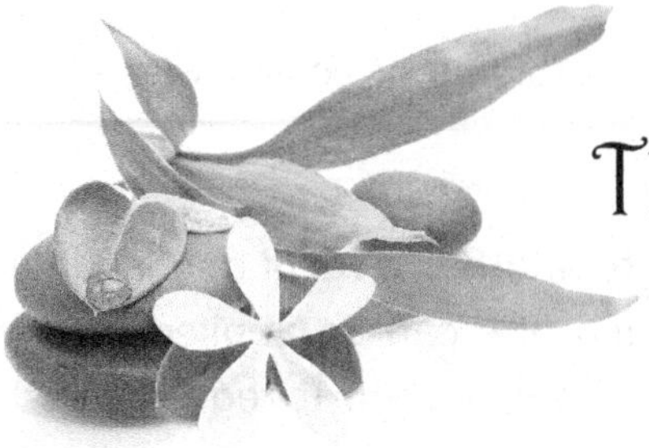

The Practice

EXERCISES FOR SELF-AWARENESS AND SELF-REGULATION

Exercise 1:
Mindfulness Practice

How can I do this exercise?

In this exercise we focus our attention on each of the Five Windows of Awareness (see below), in turn, noticing what we are experiencing in the present moment. We can do this by giving brief periods of attention to our breath, our senses, our body parts, our thoughts, feelings and our sense of interconnection, according to the instructions below. One by one, read each instruction and (apart from the one for 'sight') close your eyes briefly while you bring your awareness to that which is to be observed, for 10 to 20 seconds.

Adopt the attitude of a curious scientist, observing without judging or comparing. We'll begin with observing the breath, followed by the Five Windows of Awareness.

Breath:

- ◇ We begin with bringing our awareness to our breath:
- ◇ Notice the breath moving in and out of the nostrils.
- ◇ Notice the breath in the throat.

◇ Notice the breath in the chest.
◇ Notice the breath in the abdomen.

Window 1:

◇ Now we bring our awareness to our senses:
◇ Notice what you can taste.
◇ Notice the sensation of touch in your hands and feet where they are in contact with something.
◇ Notice any sounds you can hear.
◇ Notice what you can see (with open eyes).
◇ Notice what you can smell.

Window 2:

◇ Now we bring our awareness to our body:
◇ Notice the sensations in your hands and then arms.
◇ Notice the sensations in your feet and legs.
◇ Notice the sensations in the front of your body.
◇ Notice the sensations in the back of your body.
◇ Notice the sensations in your head.

Window 3:

◇ Now we bring our attention to our thoughts:
◇ Notice any thoughts that appear.
◇ Notice any beliefs you might have right now.
◇ Notice any assumptions you might be making right now.
◇ Notice any judgements you might be making right now.

Window 4:

◇ Now we bring our attention to our feelings:
◇ Notice any positive feeling you might have right now.

- ◇ Notice any negative feeling you might have right now.
- ◇ Notice any patience you might have right now.
- ◇ Notice any impatience you might have right now.
- ◇ Notice any happiness you might be feeling right now.
- ◇ Notice any unhappiness you might be feeling right now.
- ◇ Notice any gratitude you might be feeling right now.
- ◇ Notice any envy you might be feeling right now.

Window 5:

- ◇ Now we bring our attention to our sense of interconnection:
- ◇ Notice any sense of attunement with your mother.
- ◇ Notice any sense of attunement with your father.
- ◇ Notice any sense of attunement with your partner or best friend.
- ◇ Notice any sense of attunement with one or more of your children.
- ◇ Notice any sense of attunement with all of humanity.
- ◇ Notice any sense of attunement with Nature.
- ◇ Notice any sense of attunement with your higher Self, the real you.

<u>Exercise 2:</u>
Mindfulness Exercise: Being Present

How can I do this exercise?

Sometime during the afternoon or evening take a little time to reflect and write about what you became aware of during those moments when you were fully present. Record your observations in your journal. An entry might look like this:

Date: Friday, 15th May 2016

Today, when I stayed present to:

My senses:

"I watched a fly on my sink. I smelled the fragrance of the flowers. I listened to the sound of my coffee pot. I tasted the creamy tartness of yoghurt. I felt the changing pressures of the hard plastic scoop in my hand as I cleaned the cat's litter box."

My body:

"I observed that my body felt energetic in the morning. When I checked my body around 3 pm I observed that my neck was tight and I was thirsty."

My emotions:

"When I stopped for a while around midday, I became aware that I was feeling sad because of some bad news from the day before. I was also aware that I felt anxious about all I had to get done before driving home from work."

My thoughts:

"When I took a few moments this afternoon, I observed that my thoughts were scattered and I was not focussed. I also noticed I had a lot of worry-type thoughts. As I write this, I notice that my thoughts are becoming more positive and peaceful."

My interconnectedness:

"When I was getting my children ready for school, I was reflecting on the thoughts and feelings I have toward them. I took a moment to connect with my heart and consciously send my children heartfelt intentions of love and safety."

Exercise 3:

Mindfulness Practice: Making Room for Uncomfortable Feelings

How can I do this exercise?

- ◇ For this exercise, first you'll have to decide upon a situation that triggers an uncomfortable feeling. It might be an unpleasant memory from your own childhood or something more recent. If you don't feel that you are ready to focus on your most upsetting memory, start with something less disturbing.

Having decided on the memory, let's begin:

- ◇ Imagine first of all being in that situation again and notice what that feels like.
- ◇ Notice if the feeling is disturbing or uncomfortable.
- ◇ Now look around inside your body and see if you can tell where this uncomfortable feeling is in your body.
- ◇ Do you feel it in your head?
- ◇ Do you feel it in your stomach or your chest?
- ◇ Or do you feel it somewhere else?
- ◇ Now, pick the worst part of that uncomfortable feeling and really pay attention to it.
- ◇ Using your imagination, is the uncomfortable feeling heavy like a big stone, or is it light, like a feather?
- ◇ Does it feel like water? ... Or does it feel like a lump of clay? ... Or is it hard like wood or steel?
- ◇ Is the uncomfortable feeling moving around in your body, or does it stay in the one place?
- ◇ Is the uncomfortable feeling hot? ... Is it warm? ... Or is it cold?
- ◇ Does the unpleasant feeling in your body feel rough? ... Or does it feel smooth?
- ◇ Does the uncomfortable feeling seem like it is all squeezed up and tight inside your body?
- ◇ Now, still using your imagination, we are going to make some more

room for this feeling so that it is not so uncomfortable.

- ◇ Begin with breathing in a few long deep breaths, and let all of the air go out of your lungs as you breathe out.
- ◇ Each time you breathe in, imagine the breath going all around and through the uncomfortable feeling, making lots of room for it in your stomach and chest.
- ◇ Keep making more space for this unpleasant feeling, each time you breathe.
- ◇ Now put your hand on the part of your body where this uncomfortable feeling is.
- ◇ Imagine that your hand is giving comfort to this unpleasant feeling. It is like your hand is being a kind friend to this feeling inside.
- ◇ Now, silently in your mind, imagine talking softly and gently to this uncomfortable feeling, saying, "I can feel you there, but it is OK ... I can still drive the car, go to the shops and cook food, and anything else I want to do ... You don't feel very good, but I am making room for you, so that you have more space around you ... Soon you are going to change into a really nice feeling. I know you will."
- ◇ Now cross your hands over your chest, and put a half smile on your face.
- ◇ Think of being somewhere that makes you really happy.
- ◇ Think of someone you really love being with ... Say to them in your mind, "I love you. I love you. Thank you. Thank you."
- ◇ Now put your hands down and sit quietly for a while.

<u>Exercise 4:</u>

Self-Regulation in Daily Activities

How can I do this exercise?

At the close of any one day, answer some of the following questions in your journal:

1. How many times today did I apply the STOP method or other strategies for self-regulation?
2. How did I show empathy towards others?
3. What changes do I see in my connections with others?
4. Did I make a difference in the life of others today?
5. What positive seeds did I sow today?
6. What negative seeds did I sow today?
7. What would I like to do differently?
8. Were there any moments of deeply-felt connection between my family and me?
9. Was there a time when I felt less connected to my family?
10. How am I feeling about the state of my Peaceful Mind and Open Heart?

<u>Exercise 5:</u>
The Five Keys to a Harmonious Relationship: Visualisation

How can I do this exercise?

◇ Have within sight the five keys to a harmonious relationship, described earlier (page 61).
◇ When you have some quiet time alone you can visualise being mindful of each one of the five keys in turn. This is how to do that:
◇ Decide on a friend you can focus on in your visualisation.
◇ While imagining yourself in the company of that person – just the two of you – include some reflection on each one of the five keys, taking 3 to 5 minutes for each.
◇ Now repeat the imaginary sequence with someone else.
◇ Do it for five or six people, until all have been given this special consideration.
◇ Write in your journal any insights or observations you'd like to record.

<u>Exercise 6:</u>
The Five Keys to a Harmonious Relationship: Real-life

How can I do this exercise?

◇ Have the following five reminders (representing the five keys to a harmonious relationship) written on a card for easy reference:

Attention
Acceptance
Appreciation
Attunement
Allowing

◇ When you are alone with one of your friends, colleagues or family members (say, walking together, preparing food, working together, etc.), focus your attention on each one of the key reminders, in turn, for about 3 to 5 minutes each.

◇ Later, write in your journal any insights or observations you'd like to record.

<u>Exercise 7:</u>
Developing Resilience: The Healthy Mind Platter

How can I do this exercise?

◇ Reflect on each one of the seven practices for the Healthy Mind Platter, described earlier.
◇ Give yourself a rating of 1 to 5 to indicate the extent to which you engage in this practice.
◇ Create an action plan for increasing the amount of time that you give to the practice with the lowest rating.
◇ After a few weeks, note in your journal the effects of enacting your action plan.

<u>Exercise 8:</u>
Finding your Centre using Defusion

How can I do this exercise?

◇ Reflect on the four methods for using Defusion to let go of intrusive, disturbing thoughts, described earlier.
◇ Practise the defusion techniques on yourself, using in turn each one of:
  - Passengers on a Bus
  - Shift and Shine

- ▸ Leaves on a Stream
- ▸ STOP

<u>Exercise 9:</u>
The Five C's of Resilient Coping

How can I do this exercise?

- ◇ Spend some time reading and reflecting upon each one of the five C's for enhancing resilience:

  - ▸ Calm
  - ▸ Clarity
  - ▸ Connection
  - ▸ Competence
  - ▸ Courage

- ◇ Rate yourself 1 to 10 as to the extent to which you generally make use of each one of the five C's.
- ◇ Create an action plan for increasing the effectiveness of the lowest-rated C.

<u>Exercise 10:</u>
Relationship: Mindfully Finding the Balance

How can I do this exercise?

- ◇ Read and reflect upon each of the brain-balancing methods described earlier:

- ► Connect and redirect
- ► Name it to tame it
- ► Move the body
- ► Acts of compassion and forgiveness

◇ Practise applying one or more of these techniques to yourself, each time you feel disturbed.

◇ Note your progress in your journal.

◇ Try explaining and demonstrating each of the methods to a friend or colleague.

◇ Offer assistance to your friend or colleague by applying one of the above brain-balancing methods, the next time they become disturbed by some upsetting experience.

Your vision will become clear
only when you look into your heart.
Who looks outside dreams,
who looks inside awakens.

Carl Gustav Jung

Chapter 4

Coming Home to our Authentic Happiness

Authentic happiness refers to a rich, full and meaningful life.
When we take action on the things that truly matter
deep in our hearts, when we move in directions
that we consider valuable and worthy,
when we clarify what we stand for in life and act accordingly,
then our lives become rich and full and meaningful,
and we experience a powerful sense of vitality.
It is a profound sense of life well-lived.

Russ Harris

Most of us would agree from our own experience that, if we could live every moment of our lives feeling a peace beyond compare, one that was unaffected by whatever happens to us, we would have discovered a level of long-lasting happiness that we all yearn for. Surely unruffled equanimity and contentment – a deep abiding peace, a profound sense of wellbeing – is the most priceless possession we could ever have.

Similarly, if we could see the radiant sun of each person's spirit shining behind their clouds of fear, selfishness, desire, pride and anger, there would be a sense of intimate companionship with all whom we meet. Just recently the founder of the Hard Rock Cafe chain, Isaac Tigrett, said to an audience something like, "I am in awe at what I can see in every single person I talk to. There is such beauty, wisdom and power in there." As such, he is able to love everyone the same, loving the Love that he sees behind their eyes. Surely it would be a life well-lived if we could recognise ourselves and all others as waves on an endless sea of the highest Love.

In 2012, a pioneer in the positive psychology field, Martin Seligman published his book, *Flourish: A Visionary New Understanding of Happiness and Wellbeing,* in which he proposed that we are all inherently motivated to pursue and be engaged in five key areas of experience and behaviour, each of which contributes to our storehouse of a more authentic and long-lasting happiness. These well-researched foundations for a life that is both satisfying and fulfilling are described as follows:

❖ **P**ositive Emotions:	The enhancement of positive emotions
❖ Positive **R**elationships:	The building of positive relationships
❖ Positive **E**ngagement:	The development of social and emotional competency
❖ Positive **M**eaning:	The fostering of a sense of meaning and purpose
❖ Positive **A**ccomplishment:	The use of strength-based approaches

As can be seen in the description of authentic happiness given by Russ Harris at the start of this chapter, such an advanced level of general wellbeing is far beyond the transient pleasures that come with satisfying bodily needs (e.g. hunger), indulging the senses (e.g. watching movies) or inflating the ego (e.g. competing).

In the light of our understanding that the five universal Human Values (Love, Peace, Truth, Right Conduct and Non-violence) are inborn, we can also regard authentic happiness as our natural state, one that calls to us from within to search for and find the cave in our heart wherein it dwells. According to Martin Seligman, it calls to us through the medium of the five elements (listed above) that he has identified as pathways to a more authentic, lasting and fulfilling happiness.

We realised that the high-lighted letters in the above table spell out PREMA which is the ancient Sanskrit word for the Human Value of Love, the essence of all five of the Human Values. Based on our long-term study and application of these Values in educational, clinical and aged-care settings, it is our belief that each one of the five Positives listed above requires the involvement of pure Love for it to reach its full potential. That is, we will not be able to have genuine Positive Emotions without the inclusion or presence of the Human Value of Love. Similarly, truly Positive Relationships between ourselves and others will not be possible without the fostering of unconditional Love; and the same applies also for Positive Engagement, Positive Meaning and Positive Accomplishment. Let us explore each one of these five foundations for experiencing authentic happiness and wellbeing.

Foundation One

Positive Emotions: The enhancement of positive emotions

Saints and sages have told us throughout history that we are surrounded and saturated by a vast, limitless ocean of unalloyed bliss. The perennial philosophy of Vedanta assures us that every atom, every cell, in every human being and all of creation is made up of Sath-Chith-Ananda (Being-Awareness-Bliss). It says that, when we are aware (Chith) of our true Self (Sath), we are in a state of unsurpassed bliss (Ananda). Out of the thousand pathways for arriving at this, our natural state, perhaps one of the most important is to adopt the conviction that ongoing, unbounded, pure happiness is already within us. Without this certitude, we are at risk of being led astray by two common self-deceptions.

The first erroneous belief is that grief, anxiety and other disturbing emotions are part of who we are, instead of recognising that they are benevolent signals from our wise unconscious telling us that we have turned away from our Sun to face our shadow. That is, we have turned away from abiding by our true Self – the universal Human Values of Love, Truth, Peace, Right Conduct and Non-violence – instead of embracing It as who we really are. As an example of this approach, the Sufi poet Rumi says, "How long will you move backwards? Come forward. In grief, see gentleness; come towards gentleness."

The second error that can lead us away from our innate happiness, our Peaceful Mind and Open Heart, is a belief that love, peace and happiness only come to us through what our senses and the world can give to us. As an example, we know that those who are always yearning to be loved are bound to be unhappy, because they don't realise that they are already Love itself – as Saint Francis of Assisi said, "What you are looking for, is what is looking."

Whereas the foregoing suggestions rely upon having a reasoned faith in the wisdom of the great spiritual masters throughout history, in the past two decades there have been many research studies demonstrating that positive emotions can be generated by engaging in activities that are really aspects of the Human Values in action. For example, two of the prominent research psychologists in this area, Sonja Lyubomirsky and Martin Seligman, have shown that positive activities such as writing letters of gratitude, performing five or more kind acts every day, visualising our ideal selves, practising forgiveness and so on, all improve feelings of happiness and wellbeing.

There is real merit in the many sayings of old such as 'Always be happy', 'Do unto others as you would have them do unto you', 'Hurt never, help ever' and 'Love all, serve all'. If indeed our natural inborn state is an authentic happiness beyond measure, it makes perfect sense for us to bring the Human Value of Love into all of our activities, even going out of our way to engage in acts of kindness, friendliness, caring, compassion, helping, generosity, sharing and so on. And it also makes sense to regard all of our negative feelings as not being who we really are – like the fish when it finds itself stranded out of the water; it uses its discomfort as an incentive to find its way back into its rightful habitat.

All negative emotions originate from Fear.
And all positive emotions originate from Love.

Renee Cefalu

Foundation Two

Positive Relationships: The building of positive relationships

Research psychologists have been investigating why it is that married people live longer, are healthier and more likely to retain their mental faculties later in life, compared with those who remain single. Couples who remain united as they grow older have generally learned how to develop a positive relationship, one that is mutually supportive in facing challenges and more other-focussed than self-centred. In their 2014 study, psychologists Brook Feeney and Nancy Collins showed that, in supportive relationships, one person can help another to 'thrive' (that is, to have an increase in general happiness, positive self-regard, purpose and meaning, social wellbeing and also physical health). When we feel supported, loved, respected and accepted, we are emboldened to reach beyond our limiting concepts of who we think we are and what we can achieve; and we are better able to withstand those gale-force winds of adversity that would otherwise have overwhelmed us.

How are we to build these positive relationships? Positive psychology now has considerable research material demonstrating that learning to listen, to give help and to forgive, cooperate and unify, results in enhanced wellbeing and authentic happiness, both for the receiver and for the provider of such unconditional love. Further, those who extend their kindness, generosity, gratitude and forgiveness to everyone reap the just rewards of being much loved and supported themselves. When ex-Harvard professor, Baba Ram Dass (formerly Richard Alpert), suffered a crippling stroke in his 70's after decades of giving his all to help and inspire others, donations came pouring in from all over the world to provide for his nursing care and rehabilitation.

Our own understanding of what comes under the umbrella of 'positive relationships' includes the quality of the relationship we have with ourselves and with Nature, with animals, plants and all living and non-living things. The Human Value of Love says that we cannot have a truly positive relationship with other people without at the same time loving and respecting ourselves and the natural elements that support us. If we continue to eschew having a mutually-supportive relationship with the natural environment that does its best to care for us, the challenge of attaining local, national and global harmony, and finding authentic happiness and wellbeing in an over-heated world with denuded lands and acidic oceans, will be so much greater than it is now.

Having positive relationships with people brings us happiness. When we also love ourselves and the land, sky and sea, we surround that joy and wellbeing with a protective fence.

People will forget what you said, people will forget what you do,
but people will never forget how you made them feel.

Jason Barger

Foundation Three

Positive Engagement: Becoming fully present, intentional, in the present moment

Those working in the field of positive psychology have borrowed the word 'flow' to describe being fully engaged, with delight, in the present activity, whether it be social, work-related, family, physical, artistic, meditative or any other. 'Flow' conjures up images of a river, flowing steadily towards its destination and ultimate union (becoming one) with the ocean.

One aspect of the Human Value of Truth is its depiction of Oneness, whereby the ideal for any activity – say, painting – is for the artist, the canvas, the paint and brushes, the object being painted, and also the act of painting, to be all experienced as One. That is, the artist in the flow is no longer aware of any separation between himself, the materials, the object and the process of painting.

Secondly, to be fully engaged in the present moment, we need to practise the art of mindfulness or one-pointed attention. Unless the artist can focus on his materials, the object, the act of painting and his every breath, to the exclusion of all else, full blissful immersion in the flow will not be possible.

It is our contention that a third prerequisite is required before we can have full positive engagement, and that is for each one of the Human Values to be present also. The reason for this becomes clear when we think about someone who is unable to stop playing computer games even when the body is exhausted and ill. Certainly there is full engagement to the exclusion of all else, but there is an absence of Love, Peace, Non-violence and Right Conduct, as indicated by the lack of caring for himself and for others, the restlessness and a dearth of any lasting joy, as well as by his disregarding of conscience and of his duties to family and society.

The finest example of how to be positively engaged in our social interactions is that of the baby who looks at us with unblinking eyes alight with love and joy, without any judgment or expectation, and oblivious to all else except this heart-felt sense of Oneness in the present moment.

If we can learn to love every breath, be grateful for everything and everybody, be fully in the present moment and empower ourselves by exercising fully our prime character strengths (say, kindness and curiosity), our engagement with people and activities will be rich and fulfilling, immersing us again and again in the bliss of Oneness, of flowing with the current of the whole universe.

Live as if you were to die tomorrow.
Learn as if you were to live forever.

Mahatma Gandhi

Foundation Four

Positive Meaning: The fostering of a sense of meaning and purpose

The perennial question throughout human existence has always been, "Why am I here? What is the purpose of my being born into this human form, in this time and place, to live under these circumstances?" Recently we spoke with a man in his 60's who had cared for his recently-departed, severely-disabled wife for over 30 years. He was challenged with the thought of, "If there is a God or Higher Power, how could the grand design be so cruel that the person I loved so dearly had to endure severe physical pain and the indignity of requiring total care five times a day for all of her too-short life?" We said to him something like:

> Universal spiritual truth is beyond words, but we can approximate it by using stories, good stories, because only the good story brings joy, peace and meaning. A good story for you could be about the sugarcane: It has to be burned, slashed, crushed, boiled and dried, all so that the sweet sugar inside can be revealed. In the same way, all of our pains and disappointments come into our lives to destroy the ego barriers enclosing our true nature, our Peaceful Mind and Open Heart. You treasured being with your beloved because she was connected with her 'sweetness' within, much more than others.

Making up good stories might involve being deeply committed to a spiritual philosophy, one that gives purpose and meaning to our lives. Sayings like, 'Everything is good or leading towards the good' or the Saint Francis prayer which begins with, 'Make me an instrument of Thy peace', can be powerful reminders of a deeper purpose and meaning underlying events or actions that might not make sense to the logical mind.

Apart from making up good stories to give meaning and purpose to our lives and those of others, there are a number of research-based findings that have identified the most-important ingredients for a meaningful life. These are:

- Enjoying high-quality relationships (e.g. avoiding low-quality ones; loving others instead of seeking to be loved; fostering friendships with mutually-supportive and respectful people)
- Being helpful and kind (e.g.visiting or phoning lonely people; learning to really listen; seeking to do six kind things every day)
- Dedicating time and energy to something greater than ourselves (e.g. such as world poverty, refugees, global warming)
- Where possible, being employed in work that is consistent with our personal values and beliefs
- Integrating the five Human Values of Love, Truth, Peace, Right Conduct and Non-violence into all of our thoughts, words and actions (e.g. avoiding any that are unkind and harmful to others)

- Seeking to maximise the expression of our character strengths (e.g. bravery, by facing each one of our fears and learning to like our dislikes; or love of learning, by mastering new skills)

When we have such purpose and meaning in our lives, we are no longer constrained by procrastination, timidity, doubt and uncertainty. We can now turn towards our unfolding destiny with a passion for life, enjoying an authentic happiness and wellbeing that is denied to us when we are drifting like a boat in a vast open sea.

Learn to light a candle in the darkest moments of someone's life.
Be the light that helps others see; it is what gives life
its deepest significance.

Roy T. Bennett

Foundation Five

Positive Accomplishment: The use of strength-based approaches

If we were to wonder, "When does a tree on a mountain feel the most joy in accomplishment?" we might conclude that it's when fierce winds are blowing, prompting the tree to send stabilising roots down deeper into the ground, wherein it finds more water and nutrients for it to grow stronger and taller.

And if we were to ask whether an ant, a bee, a fish or a butterfly feels a special happiness when achieving something truly great and beautiful, we can imagine that they do, because every part of Nature is responding to that inner call to exercise the talents and skills that are uniquely theirs.

The nature of fire is to burn and that of water to quench thirst; that of the sun is to sacrifice itself to provide light and heat to us all; and that of the stars at night is to remind us that the darker the night, the brighter the light. Every part of Nature is following its inner blueprint that defines its dutiful activities, using their innate skills for the good of all, and in doing so, teaching us how to live lovingly, wisely, selflessly, powerfully and beautifully.

Developmental psychologists and neuroscientists affirm that, particularly during our early formative years, our brain is hard-wired to accomplish great things. Armed only with great perseverance and cheerful determination, without any encouragement or extrinsic rewards, each one of us as a young child created and programmed specialised neuronal circuits in our brain to give us control over fine and gross motor movements, speech, memory, discrimination and thinking. Given a multi-lingual environment, even impoverished young children readily learn to understand and speak two or more languages, all in the absence of any structured teaching programs.

How did we manage to achieve all of this? As with every living thing in Nature, we obeyed those inner promptings that conveyed "Do this" and, beginning with the most minute of movements, we steadily built upon the more solid of the foundations we had laid down for each component of a skill until success and then even more success was achieved.

Positive psychology proposes that in adulthood we can follow an identical formula for gaining authentic happiness and wellbeing through what we accomplish. Psychologists Martin Seligman and Chris Peterson, leaders in the positive psychology movement, have identified 24 character strengths (e.g. creativity, perseverance, kindness, fairness, forgiveness, gratitude, and so on) that fall under six broad virtue categories: wisdom, courage, humanity, justice, temperance and transcendence. These 24 strengths describe the range of personality traits that exist in people across all countries and cultures. They describe our capacities for helping ourselves and others, and we feel good when we put them into action. Our Signature Strengths are those character strengths that stand out in our lives, the ones we feel best about and that others observe in us. To identify your top strengths, go to www.via.character.org or do the quiz on psychologist Martin Seligman's Authentic Happiness website. Researchers in positive psychology advise us that, if we are to experience a more lasting happiness and wellbeing, it would be best to ensure that all of our activities incorporate our Signature Strengths so that we are motivated to be fully engaged in what we do.

At the beginning of this chapter, we proposed that, with the Human Value of Love running as a current through all of the elements in the acronym PRE-MA (Positive Emotions, Positive Relationships, and so on), they can be seen as pathways towards realising our higher Self, towards living and breathing our true nature, the five Human Values, our Peaceful Mind and Open Heart, towards embracing the authentic happiness that is our birthright.

To the extent that we can apply the principles of PREMA, while doing our best to live the Human Values in every moment, our advancing years will be rich and fulfilling in this university of life. Then, as we move into our closing years, we'll be ready for the post-graduate studies that lead up to our final graduation, all of which build upon the bedrock of love and wisdom laid down in the preceding years.

All that is sweet, delightful, and amiable in this world,
in the serenity of the air, the fineness of seasons,
the joy of light, the melody of sounds, the beauty of colours,
the fragrance of smells, the splendour of precious stones,
is nothing else but Heaven
breaking through the veil of this world,
manifesting itself in such a degree and
darting forth in such variety so much of its own nature.

William Law

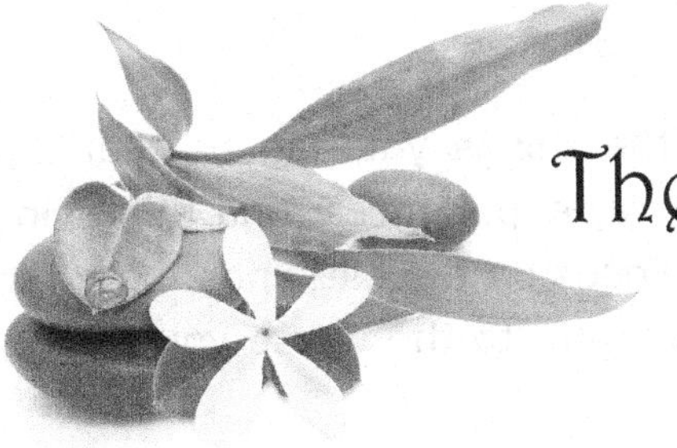

The Practice

EXERCISES TO CULTIVATE POSITIVITY IN OUR LIFE

<u>Exercise 1:</u>
Expressing Gratitude

How can I do this exercise?

There are a number of simple activities we can engage in to increase and cultivate an attitude of gratitude.

◇ Give sincere thanks to others.

When someone does something to make our day happier or easier, we can be quick to verbalize our thanks and appreciation. Not only will it make the person feel good, it will give us a wave of happiness too. It's an instant reward to see how expressing gratitude makes a positive difference in someone else's day. It makes us realize that we're all connected and that what we do matters.

◇ Keep a gratitude journal.

Write down the good things that happened to you during the day. Research shows that keeping a gratitude journal is a powerful technique that instantly makes us feel happier, more connected to others and genuinely appreciative.

◇ Count your blessings.

Make it a habit to reflect on the things you can be thankful for. Bring to mind all the good people, experiences, and things in your life, both now and in the past. Focus on the blessings, both big and small, from the people who love you, to the house you live in, and the food on your table.

◇ Write a letter of gratitude.

Think of someone who did something that changed your life for the better, someone you never properly thanked. Write a thoughtful letter of gratitude expressing what the person did, how it affected you, and what it still means to you. Then deliver the letter.

◇ Find the positive in a negative event from the past.

Even the most painful circumstances can teach us positive lessons. We can re-evaluate a negative event from our past with an eye for what we learned or how we became stronger, wiser, or more compassionate.

<u>Exercise 2:</u>
Nurture and Enjoy Relationships

How can I do this exercise?

◇ Make a conscious effort to stay connected.

Make an effort to stay connected to the people who make your life brighter. Take the time to call, write, or arrange to see each other in person.

◇ Invest in quality time with the people you care about.

It is not just the time spent with friends and family that matters; it is how we spend it. People who are in happy relationships share a lot. They share what's going on in their lives and how they feel. Follow their example and carve out time to talk and enjoy each other's company.

◇ Offer sincere compliments.

Think of the things you admire and appreciate about the other person and then tell them. As a practice of gratitude, it will make you value the relationship more and feel happier.

◇ Seek out happy people.

Make an effort to seek out and spend time with happy people.

◇ Take delight in the good fortune of others.

Show genuine enthusiasm and interest when your friend or family member experiences something good. Ask questions, relive the experience with the other person, and express your excitement for him or her.

Exercise 3:

Live in the Moment and Savour Life's Pleasures

How can I do this exercise?

- ◇ Be mindful and fully engaged in the here-and-now.

  There are a number of mindfulness exercises in Part Four that help us focus on the present moment, so we can feel more balanced, happy and at peace (pages 223 - 232).

- ◇ Adopt enjoyable daily rituals.

  Build moments of enjoyment into your day with pleasurable rituals. These can be very simple things like lingering over a cup of coffee in the morning, taking a short stroll in the sunshine during our lunch hour, or playing with our dog when we get home.

- ◇ Minimize multi-tasking.

  Focus on one thing at a time in order to truly maximize your attendance to and enjoyment in what you are doing.

- ◇ Stop to smell the roses.

  Stop whatever you're doing for a moment to appreciate and luxuriate in your surroundings. It will enhance your pleasure, even if you can only spare a few seconds. Sometimes you can share the moment with others.

- ◇ Replay happy memories.

  Remembering and reminiscing about happy memories and experiences from our past leads to more positive emotions in the present.

Exercise 4:

Focus on Helping Others and Living with Meaning

How can I do this exercise?

◇ Practise kindness.

Look for ways to be more kind, compassionate and giving in your daily life. This can be something as small as brightening a stranger's day with a smile or going out of our way to do a favour for a friend.

◇ Use our strengths for the greater good.

There are many different kinds of strengths, including kindness, curiosity, honesty, creativity, love of learning, perseverance, loyalty, optimism and other virtues that can be used for the greater good.

◇ Be in the flow.

Flow happens when we're actively engaged in something that is intrinsically rewarding and challenging, yet still attainable. Anything that completely captivates us and engages our full attention can be a flow activity.

◇ Volunteer.

You will get the most out of the experience of volunteering by joining an organization that you believe in and that allows you to contribute in a meaningful way.

Exercise 5:
Take Better Care of Health

How can I do this exercise?

◇ Make exercise a regular habit.

Exercise is good for the body and also has a powerful effect on mental wellbeing.

◇ Get the sleep you need.

Getting quality sleep every night directly affects our happiness, vitality, and emotional stability during the day. According to sleep scientists, the average person needs at least 6 to 9 hours each night.

Exercise 6:
Be Our Best Possible Selves

How can I do this exercise?

◇ Think about your best possible self.

This means that you imagine yourself in the future, after everything has gone as well as it possibly could. Imagine you have worked hard and succeeded in accomplishing all of your goals. Think of this as the realization of your life's dreams, and of your best potential.

In all of these imaginings, you are identifying the best possible way that things might turn out in your life. Doing this will make it easier for you to make good decisions now about your life's direction.

◇ Write down the ideal life that you would like to have in the future.

May our heart's garden of awakening
bloom with hundreds of flowers.

Thich Nhat Hanh

Part Two

The Role of Neuroscience in Authentic Happiness

Genuine happiness is being
in a deep sense of fulfilment
that arises from
an exceptionally healthy mind;
a way of being that pervades
all emotional states,
and gives us the inner resources
to deal with whatever comes our way.

Matthieu Ricard

Chapter 5

The Blossoming of Human Excellence in the Brain

I believe that the greatest truths of the universe
don't lie outside, in the study of the stars and the planets. They lie
deep within us, in the magnificence of our heart,
mind and soul. Until we understand what is within,
we can't understand what is without.

Anita Moorjani

Aristotle wrote that there is only one desire – the desire for happiness – and that all other desires are for the means by which that happiness might be found. Positive psychology equates supreme, lasting, undiluted happiness with what Martin Seligman calls 'authentic happiness and wellbeing', which is sought after through PREMA (Positive Emotions, Positive Relationships, Positive Engagement, Positive Meaning and Positive Accomplishment).

In the previous chapter we reasoned that the higher realms of authentic happiness can only be reached if we commit ourselves to living the five Human Values of Love, Peace, Truth, Right Conduct and Non-violence as best we can. When these universal pinnacles of good character saturate and direct our lives, the five elements of PREMA (emotions, relationships, engagement, meaning and accomplishment) will not be impeded in their flowering by human frailties such as fear, pride, selfishness and attachments. Then we can be liberated from littleness into vastness, from fear-driven limitation to boundless, lasting, unalloyed happiness. Such is our potential, our birthright, our destiny, each one of us.

Such a blossoming of human excellence does not happen without effort. It takes effort to find and extract the diamond from the core of the mountain, and it takes effort to chip and wash away the dirt and stones still clinging to its pristine surface. The end result of such sustained endeavour is its own reward – the blossoming of human excellence, the experience of expansion, inclusiveness, selflessness, lasting joy and satisfaction.

The Brain and the Mind

All of this evolution in thinking, feeling and behaving is intimately involved with the brain. Our brain is the most important organ in our body, and what happens in it determines what we think and feel, say and do. What flows through our mind sculpts our brain. Thus, we can use our mind to change our brain for the better, and this in turn will improve our mind – which will benefit our whole being, and every other person whose life we touch.

Modern medicine, neuropsychiatry and clinical psychology have been demonstrating for over fifty years how greatly the mind depends on the brain. For example, as the brain develops in childhood, so does the mind; if the brain is ever damaged, so is the mind; subtle shifts in brain chemistry will alter mood, concentration, and memory.

We experience our greatest happiness, our deepest peace, our most fulfilling love and our most satisfying activity when our mind becomes still, when we experience the state of no-mind, unwavering mind or thought-less awareness. In this state our mind has given its allegiance to the heart and willingly takes up residence in that abode.

Neurophysiological and neurobiochemical researchers have also coined the terms transcendental mind, restful alertness and transcendental consciousness to describe this condition of the mind, delineating it from the ordinary waking, sleeping and dreaming states.

Research studies indicate that, when the mind is still, there is increased mental alertness and this is accompanied by the mobilization of hidden reserves in the brain that enliven brain functioning over a wide area. In short, we can say that, when the body/mind complex is in a condition of Peaceful Mind, Open Heart, our memory, discrimination, decision-making and mental alertness are all increased. That is, we move closer to experiencing our innate human excellence to the extent that we can practise mindful awareness where the mind is alert and resting in the cave of the heart.

Of course we know from our own experience that the mind is not able to relinquish its hold on the world and be still while we remain locked up in the prison created by the mind. The prison is, firstly, the belief that we are this body, mind and feelings rather than the ever-present Witness of these changing scenes; and secondly, the assumption that happiness is granted to us through the satisfaction of our wants and needs, rather than it being ever-present within us in boundless abundance. Letting go of these misinformed beliefs is an essential pre-requisite for giving the Heart and Soul sovereignty over the mind; and this is followed by the even greater challenge of remembering to do so.

There is a useful metaphor for describing this ongoing 'work' that is required of us if we are to live in accordance with our inborn human excellence. It is that of a coach that has a driver sitting up top using the reins to control the horses. The coach represents the body; the horses are the senses and emotions; the driver is our intellect or discriminating function; the reins are the mind; and the passenger inside the coach is our true Self. In the general human condition, the passenger (the true Self) is 'asleep' inside the coach (the body), leaving the driver (the intellect) without any guidance as to the destination (Peaceful Mind, Open Heart; no mind; human excellence). As such, the reins (our mind) are not utilised to exert control over the horses (senses and emotions), leaving us at the mercy of whatever whim or fancy is foremost.

Saints and sages and the founders of the major religions (e.g. Jesus, Buddha, Krishna, Zoroaster) have all advised us in different ways that we need to use the mind to get rid of the mind, in the same way that we use a thorn to dislodge another thorn embedded in the foot. The challenge is to 'wake up', again and again, so as to ensure that the intellect is not allowing the senses and emotions to have free rein. We 'wake up' each time we return our attention to the breath, or repeat a prayer or affirmation, or put a ceiling on how much we indulge a desire, or let go of a distracting thought or disturbing emotion, or be one-pointed in focussing our attention on a leaf or a candle flame. The Russian-Armenian mystic G. I. Gurdjieff used to remind his students to 'remember to remember that you are asleep'. It is a challenge for us all to find ways of reminding ourselves that most of the time we forget that we are operating in automatic mode, like a pre-programmed robot: habitually focussing our attention on the past or the future instead of the present; making judgments, blaming or criticising instead of seeing the perfection in every moment; or reacting with fear and avoidance when something challenges us to 'wake up'.

Sathya Sai Baba often gave wrist watches to people, along with the advice to refer to the acronym of WATCH whenever they could remember to do so. That is:

Watch your **W**ords
Watch your **A**ctions
Watch your **T**houghts
Watch your **C**haracter
Watch your **H**eart

Each time we remember to be mindful in this or in any other way, we are reinforcing a set of neural pathways in the brain that makes it more likely that we will remember to WATCH - to be more aware or mindful of ourselves.

As noted earlier, the brain not only provides the necessary infrastructure for the functioning of the mind, it is also influenced and shaped by the mind that it supports. This is how skills, habits, fears, preferences and attitudes are developed: through the activity of the mind as it creates and reinforces specific clusters of neural pathways in the brain.

Our experiences matter, not just for how they feel in the moment, but for the lasting traces they leave in our brain. All occasions of rich and prolonged contentment, happiness, awe, enthusiasm, humility, selfless love, or any other ideal state can make real changes in our neural networks. The structure-building processes of the nervous system are turbocharged by conscious experience, and especially by what is in the foreground of our awareness.

The scale of the brain's operation is beyond comprehension. The brain's tofu-like tissue contains 1.1 trillion *cells*, including 100 billion *neurons*. Each neuron can receive an average of about five thousand connections, called *synapses,* from other neurons. When activated, a typical neuron fires 5 to 50 times a second, sending bursts of chemicals, called *neurotransmitters,* to other neurons. While you are reading one line of this page, perhaps 100 million neurons in your brain are firing off in highly integrated circuits. The number of possible combinations of neural signals in our brain at any given moment is estimated to far exceed the number of atoms in the whole universe.

Each firing of a neuron is a bit of information. We now know that our nervous system moves information around like our heart moves blood around. All of that information is what is broadly defined as *mind*, most of which remains outside of our awareness. So we can see that the scale and scope of the human mind is so vast and powerful that we cannot put a limit on what it is capable of.

Given the near-infinite potential of the mind/brain connections, we can readily accept that, by following certain procedures over time, a human being can grow the number of lasting neural circuits required for each one of the universal Human Values to be manifested constantly; that is, for us to be in an unbroken state of pure Love and untold bliss, with access to the wisdom of the sages and all possible knowledge. We can even imagine (indeed, propose) that it is possible to program the mind to remain focussed every moment on that unchanging aspect of ourselves that is ever-witnessing all of our thoughts, words and deeds (in the same way that the movie screen is constantly aware of the images projected onto its surface, yet remains untouched, unaffected by their presence or absence).

In other words, as the mystics, saints and sages have reminded us throughout history, we can learn to live in such a way as to be unaffected by whatever calamity befalls the body through life.

Habits and the Brain

In recent years neuroscience has been giving us tangible evidence that, to develop any advanced skills – such as the blossoming of human excellence – we need to apply repetition, struggle, perseverance and effort so as to build super-fast neural pathways in the brain that will enable that skill to become an ingrained habit. Such neural networks will give priority to the enactment of desired behaviours, rather than allow distractions from any source. Let us look at this in more detail.

At the beginning of this century a new technology called diffusion tensor imaging allowed brain scientists to create computer-generated images of *myelinated* circuits within the living human brain. Myelin is a microscopic sheath that forms around neurons' axons (the end part of the neuron's stem) when a neuronal circuit is *repeatedly activated.* This sheath increases conduction speed from one neuron to another neuron across the synapse by up to a 100 times, and reduces refractory (resting) times between the firing neurons by up to 30 times, resulting in 3000 times more efficiency in that neuronal circuit in the brain.

Daniel Coyle in his 2009 book *The Talent Code* shares his insights about myelin and skills: "Skill is myelin insulation that wraps neural circuits and that grows according to certain signals." People who have developed high level skills – whether in science, mountain climbing, meditation or teaching children – all agree that things that appear to be obstacles turn out to be beneficial in due course. It seems clear that facing obstacles – instead of avoiding them – is a fundamental requirement for developing human excellence, whether it be in the field of scholasticism, physical dexterity or manifesting human excellence in our lives, Coyle says:

> *Struggle is not optional – it is neurologically required: in order to get your skill circuit to fire optimally, you must by definition fire the circuit suboptimally; you must make mistakes and pay attention to those mistakes; you must slowly teach your circuit. You must also keep firing that circuit – i.e. practising, in order to keep myelin functioning properly. After all, myelin is living tissue.*

This finding has important implications for those wanting to establish the neural circuits for human excellence in the brain. Those of us who struggle, make mistakes and lose the motivation to keep going can be inspired to change our attitude - to regard mistakes as not only 'inputs of essential information' but also the rocket fuel for advanced skill development. Although perseverance can be uncomfortable at first, it is helpful for us to know that 'pushing on' is also a skill to be developed and that, each time we try once more, because of myelin it gets easier to persevere.

When we are committed to becoming all that we can be, it is important to be reminded that every distraction or slipping back that appears to impede our progress is actually a gift, provided there is no turning away from facing the storm yet again. Of course, each one of us already knows this (about skill development), albeit at a sub-conscious level, for we were once crawling babies who, in trying to stand up and then walk, fell over perhaps 200 to 1,000 times. Thanks to myelin, each time we persevered and tried again, our skill level rose significantly. Of course at that innocent age we did not have the concepts of failure, self-doubt, or negative comparison with those already walking. Something within us welcomed the difficulty, thrived on it. Recognising this fact, we can regard all of our failures to attain unbroken equanimity and pure love as essential for our growth and turn towards these high goals with renewed faith and perseverance.

An implication of Daniel Coyle's reports and insights about myelin and accelerated learning is that setting a very high standard for ourselves – as does Ron Berger in his 2003 book, *An Ethic of Excellence* – necessarily involves embracing mistakes, setting the bar higher each time so that the mountain might appear, to the logical mind, to be impossible to climb. As Coyle says: "The trick is to choose a goal just beyond your present abilities; to target the struggle ... Allowing yourself to make mistakes, to seem stupid, makes you smarter."

The really important message from neuroscience is that plasticity – the capacity to change in response to social and physical conditions – is a core feature of the brain throughout life. That is, the brain changes in both structure and function through interactions with the environment. Two recent books by Norman Doidge, *The Brain That Changes Itself* and *The Brain's Way of Healing*, give many striking examples of how these findings are impacting in different fields of study.

Knowing that the brain can be sculptured by our experience impels us to ensure that every aspect of our life – the character of the people we spend time with; how we treat others; the recreation we engage in; how often and how earnestly we pray; whether we can persevere and be resilient during difficult times; and so on – is conducive to our brains 'growing' in optimal ways, laying the foundations for the emergence of high levels of humility, detachment, self-discipline, love, happiness and inner stillness.

The principal activities of brains are making
changes in themselves.
Marvin L. Minsky

The Ever-present Witness in the Brain

The neuropsychologists Rick Hanson and Richard Mencius, in their 2009 book *Buddha Brain: The Practical Neuroscience of Happiness, Love and Wisdom*, have brought together a number of research studies revealing that something transcendental (outside of the body) is involved with the mind, consciousness and what they call the *path of awakening*. They define this path as having the central activities of:

- ◇ The ability to reduce any stress or dysfunction
- ◇ The skill to increase wellbeing and
- ◇ The competence to support spiritual practice

This transcendental entity or presence has been called Higher Self, Spirit, Buddha nature, the Ground, the Universe, or by no name at all. In his 2012 book, *The Emotional Life of Your Brain*, psychiatrist Richard Davidson lends support to this notion that our true nature is immortal, that we do not die when the body dies and that we were not born when the baby was conceived and later born. Whatever the Soul or Buddha nature is, it is beyond the physical universe. It's presence in the body gives us a life-long opportunity to identify with it as the eternal Witness and not to identify with the body, mind and their functions. The word *enlightenment* is often used to describe having a constant awareness of and identification with this presence, this eternal Witness.

In 2002, using brain imaging techniques in their research, Andrew Newberg and Eugene d'Aquili discovered that the human brain is already hardwired for enlightenment, for rediscovering our true Self, our human excellence or Peaceful Mind, Open Heart. For example, it seems that the brain, over millions of years of evolution, has been prepared for the experience of unity with the Cosmos, with the All. Let us examine this idea in more detail.

The image Newberg captured showed that the brain's pre-frontal cortex during deep meditation (thought-less awareness) lit up in red colour, indicating an increase in blood flow and neural activity in that area. At the same time, surprisingly, the upper rear part of the brain (the parietal area) turned to a dark blue shade, indicating a sudden drop of brain activity in that area which Newberg calls the Orientation Association Area (OAA).

The OAA is the area which gives us the ability to orient ourselves in space and time and which gives our bodies a sense of physical limits and the self a sense of separateness from the rest of the universe. When the OAA is deactivated, the physical limits of the body and the sense of separateness disappears. The brain can no longer create a boundary between self and the outside world, or locate itself in physical reality. As a result, Newberg says, the brain has no choice but to perceive that self as endless, interwoven with everyone and everything. This is the state Newberg calls Absolute Unitary Being. We prefer to call it the state of Oneness.

Newberg's research suggests that the process of awakening (to the state of Oneness or human excellence) is not only due to psychological change or a change in philosophy and values. It appears to be due primarily to a fundamental change in brain function with a shift in brain dominance from the parietal (OAA) to frontal lobes of the brain (referred to by Newberg as the Attention Association Area or AAA) as in the Figure to follow. When the over-activity in the OAA is decreased and the under-activity in the AAA is increased, there is a shift of the brain's command center and the individual wakes up to a higher level of consciousness and to a new reality which seems to be even more real than the old one.

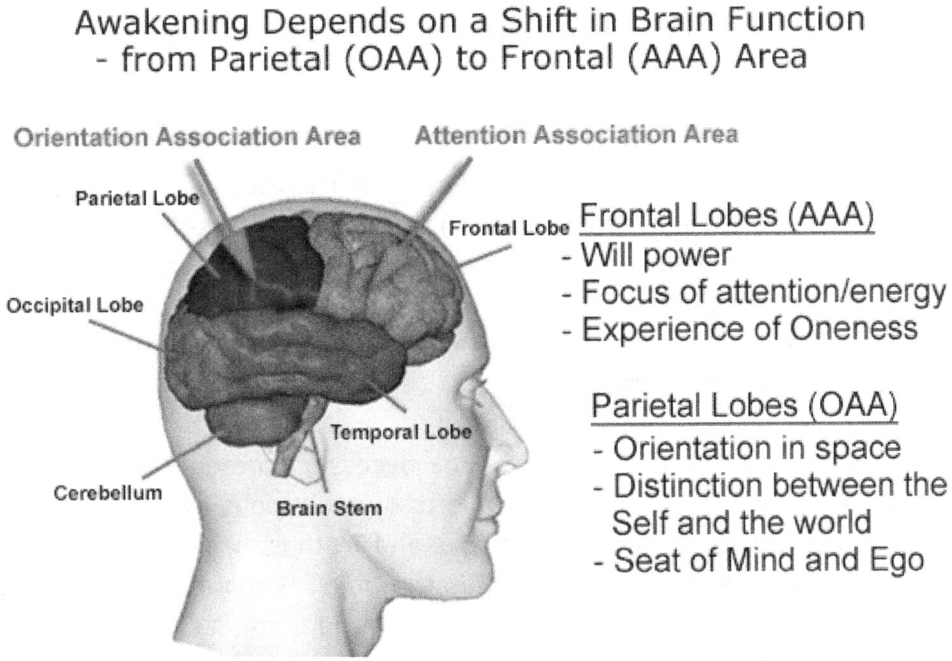

Figure: Orientation Association Area and Attention Association Area (Newberg, A., & d'Aquili, E. 2002)

Through dedicated practice in letting go of identification with the body and becoming detached from all that we have been clinging to (our various wants and desires), increasingly we are able to live every moment according to the five Human Values of Love, Peace, Truth, Right Conduct and Non-violence; that is, Peaceful Mind, Open Heart.

Each one of the Human Values is predicated upon the Truth that all is One, in the same sense that we are all waves of energy on the one vast, limitless ocean of energy that is the Cosmos. All religions and teachers of the esoteric have said that this endless ocean of energy is Love, pure sweet Love. Right Conduct is being so in tune with the one organising power of the universe that all of our activities are infused with and guided by Love, by our awareness of Oneness. Where there is perfect Love, Peace is also present because we are ever-content, being aware of our unity with all (we cannot want that which we already are, in Oneness); and, when we have a loving understanding of the perfection and interconnectedness of all things, there is Non-violence (since we are in all, there is no wish to cause harm to others in our thoughts, words or deeds).

As human beings, we are being assisted in our endeavour to experience our human excellence by a highly-evolved brain that facilitates the building of specialised neural networks in the frontal lobes, particularly the pre-frontal cortex, ones that allow us to let go of our sense of separateness and experience the reality (according to both nuclear physicists and the mystics) that there is only the Oneness.

The experience of Truth (Oneness) is the necessary prerequisite for Love at its highest level to be made available to our conscious awareness. This interdependent relationship between Love and Truth is made clearer by the metaphor: 'Truth is the current. Love is the bulb'. Without the current of Truth flowing, the Love immanent in every cell and atom in our bodies cannot shine forth. Similarly, unless we are relating from the heart, no amount of wisdom will be of any value to us.

The pre-frontal cortex appears to be the part of the brain playing the most crucial role in opening the doorways to the inner treasure of Love and the other four Human Values. When we meditate – practise mindfulness – it is as if the pre-frontal cortex is suffused with Truth through the influx of additional blood into the frontal lobes, and the reduction of blood in the parietal lobes (the agents for the illusion of separateness).

We might assume from the foregoing that every time we choose yet again to follow the path of awakening (that is, to think loving thoughts, exercise our will and restraint, practise being mindful of the present moment, follow the conscience, speak gently, be patient and forbearing, return the attention to the breath, face another fear, create order, and any of the thousand other steps on the Path), we are 'growing' the pre-frontal cortex. We are creating hundreds of millions of extra neurons and expanding those neural networks to open more doorways for the Human Values to blossom, and at the same time we are developing the skill to transfer blood from the back of the brain to the front so as to provide nutrients for added neural networks there to flourish.

The same stream of life that runs through my veins
night and day runs through the world and dances
in rhythmic measures. It is the same life that shoots
in joy through the dust of the earth in numberless
blades of grass, and breaks into tumultuous waves of
leaves and flowers. It is the same life that is rocked
in the ocean-cradle of birth and of death,
in ebb and in flow. I feel my limbs are made glorious
by the touch of this world of life.
And my pride is from the life-throb of ages
dancing in my blood this moment.

Rabindranath Tagore

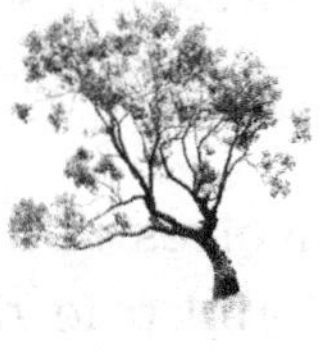

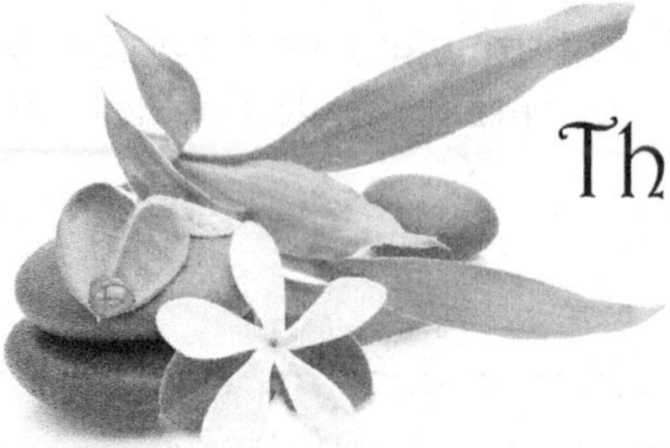

The Practice

EXERCISES FOR THE BLOSSOMING OF
HUMAN EXCELLENCE IN THE BRAIN

Exercise 1:
Contemplating on the Brain and Human Excellence

How can I do this exercise?

◇ Take a few minutes to reflect on these key points about how the brain can be 'grown' to foster the blossoming of human excellence:

- What happens in our mind changes our brain, both temporarily and in lasting ways. Therefore, we can use our mind to change our brain to benefit our mind and everyone else whose life we touch.

- The path of awakening involves both transforming the mind/brain and uncovering our wonderful true nature, our human excellence, that was there all along.

- Ordinary everyday activities – as well as any personal growth or spiritual practices – contain dozens of opportunities to change our brain from the inside out. We really do have the power, which is a wonderful thing in a world full of forces beyond our control. A single raindrop doesn't have much effect, but if we have enough raindrops and enough time, we can carve out a vast canyon.

Exercise 2:
Expanding the Mind into Oneness: The Circle

How can I do this exercise?

◇ This short exercise in imagination was popular with the great spiritual teacher, Swami Vivekananda. It involves imagining a special circle.

◇ Read the instruction first, committing it to memory, then close your eyes and imagine.

◇ Imagine you are a circle. The circumference of this circle is nowhere, and the centre of this circle is everywhere.

◇ Do this for two minutes, three times during the day, for two days.

◇ Repeat the exercise every week.

Exercise 3:
Expanding the Mind into Oneness: The Water Bubble

How can I do this exercise?

◇ This short exercise involves imagining being a water bubble on the surface of the ocean.

◇ Read the instruction first, committing it to memory, then close your eyes and imagine.

◇ Imagine you are a water bubble on the surface of the ocean; then imagine that you burst, realising now that you are the entire ocean.

◇ Repeat this imaginary sequence several times for two to five minutes, three times during the day, for two days.

◇ Repeat the exercise every week.

Exercise 4:
Expanding the Mind into Oneness: Using Light

How can I do this exercise?

◇ This exercise can take about ten minutes and is excellent for developing the feeling of oneness with everyone and everything.

◇ Read the instructions first, committing some or all of them to memory (approximately), then close your eyes and imagine.

◇ Imagine a ball of light travelling throughout your whole body, illuminating all around as it goes, until your whole body is filled with light. This can take about five minutes.

◇ Now imagine a ball of light travelling out from your heart centre (the chest) to someone you love, and see them become filled with light.

◇ Then imagine a ball of light entering more and more people, filling them with light, until everyone in the world is filled with light.

- ◇ Now imagine balls of light entering and illuminating every animal, every bird, every insect, every bush, every tree, every drop of water, every grain of sand, every molecule of air, every planet, every galaxy, until all there is, is light. Everywhere there is a vast, limitless ocean of light.

- ◇ Now say to yourself, "The light is in me. I am in the light. I am the light, everywhere," and dissolve yourself into the endless light.

- ◇ Do this every day, in the morning or before sleep, as often as you like.

<u>Exercise 5:</u>

Expanding the Mind into Oneness: Nature

How can I do this exercise?

- ◇ This exercise gradually and gently develops a feeling of love and connection with all of Nature, and even the house you live in.

- ◇ Place yourself in any of the following situations and say a few times to yourself (or out loud) , "I am in all. All are in me," and let your imagination do the rest:

- ▸ looking at the vastness of the night sky, a bird, a butterfly, a flowering bush, a tree, a sunset, or lightning flashing;

- ▸ walking through a park, in a busy street or alongside a river or stream;

- ▸ sitting in a room of your house.

◇ Do this for 2 to 5 minutes, several times every day for a week, then again after a month.

The ideals which have lighted my way,
and time after time have given me
new courage to face life cheerfully, have
been kindness, beauty and truth.

Albert Einstein

Chapter 6

The Brain, Emotions and Learning

To a mind that is still the whole universe surrenders

Lao Tzu

Throughout our lives we have been learning; learning a multitude of simple and complex skills for interacting with the world; and learning how to become master of our mind, body and emotions on our pathway of awakening to our true Self, to our innate Human Values of Love, Peace, Truth, Right Conduct and Non-violence. Modern research confirms that we learn best when our mind is steady and our emotions in balance. When we have enough passion and at the same time can be sufficiently nonchalant; when the sympathetic nervous system is not accelerating things too much and the parasympathetic nervous system is not applying the brakes too hard; and when the inhibition from our pre-frontal cortex and arousal from the limbic system in the brain are balancing each other; then we are creating some of the ideal conditions for learning. Whether we are learning how to speak a language, cook a meal or take another step towards experiencing our innate Peaceful Mind, Open Heart, the doors are held open for us if we find this inner balance.

The mind can be balanced by practising mindfulness, repeating a mantra or prayer, exploring the opposite of our fixed beliefs, and standing back from our thoughts by remembering to remember that we are the ever-present Witness of our thoughts and not the thoughts themselves. When our mind is in balance, we are in a position to use the mind to change the brain so that the mind can more readily change to support us on our journey through life.

The challenge with regulating the emotions at first seems to be far more difficult than developing some control over our mind, partly because they have been involved with our physical survival during the evolution of the human race from single-cell entities over the past 3.5 billion years. As Rick Hanson writes in *Buddha's Brain*, we have the earliest-developed 'reptilian' part of the brain sitting underneath the more recently-evolved 'mammalian' brain – the former readying us to 'fight or flee', and the latter ensuring that we can increase our chances of survival by being part of a harmonious same-species group (Handson & Mencius, 2009).

Both of these brains, each with its highly complex supporting and interactive systems (see below), are necessary for us to travel on our pathway of awakening to our inborn human excellence. We need the lower brain to motivate us to look for our inner Treasure (like a drowning man desperate to get his head up out of the water), as well as the upper, more-evolved brain which allows itself to be moulded by the mind so that it can better assist the mind to travel on this path of awakening to rediscover our true Self. It is our emotions that provide the signals as to whether we are going the right way, and also the rocket fuel for propelling us along our journey. And it is the brain that determines which emotions will come to the fore. Let us look now in a little more detail at some of what neuroscientists have been discovering about the brain, mind, emotions and learning.

Research into the brain has been accelerating at an exponential rate over the past forty years, giving us important information that impacts on how we learn, interact, find happiness and adapt. The ability of the brain to change both its functions and structure is surprisingly high – referred to as *brain plasticity*. Modifying the way we think and what we feed in through the five sense organs can assist the brain to grow in such a way that facilitates the development of human excellence.

Basic Facts of our Brain

- Any experience causes neurons in our brains to fire. Repeated experiences cause neurons to fire repeatedly. Neurons that 'fire together, wire together', strengthening neural connections.

- The *brain stem* regulates the internal homeostasis of the body (heart rate, respiratory rate, digestion, etc.) through the autonomic nervous system (ANS). The ANS has two branches, the sympathetic nervous system (SNS) for arousal and the parasympathetic (PNS) for calming.

- The *limbic region* plays an essential role in the complex cortical functions of emotional regulation and empathy, which are essential to our having understanding and to the changing patterns of attachment.

  An important part of the limbic system that influences attachment is the *amygdala*. It generates the 'fight, flight, freeze or faint' (the four F's) response by assessing every experience, including relational experience, for safety or danger, for pleasure or pain, and pairs each experience with an emotional valence (an emotional charge, positive or negative) that makes one approach or avoid similar experiences in the future.

- The *hypothalamus* is located deep in the limbic system. It releases many different hormones to regulate the amygdala. An important one is oxytocin, the bonding hormone that is released through touch, warmth and movement. Oxytocin calms the amygdala. It can spur the *pre-frontal cortex* to grow special fibres for carrying GABA (gamma butyric acid) down to the amygdala so as to quell the fear response.

- The two *hippocampi (hippocampus)*, situated on each side of the temporal lobe near the ears, are part of the limbic system. As they mature at about 2½ years of age, they begin translating experience into explicit memory, a vital part of cortical functioning. With conscious processing, one begins to remember one's experiences, including relational experiences, from 2 ½ to 3 years of age onwards.

- The *cerebral cortex* has many lobes specializing in many complex functions; these functions must be integrated for healthy relational functioning. The frontal lobes are positioned at the front-most region of the cerebral cortex and are involved in movement, decision-making, problem solving, and planning. The three main divisions of the frontal lobes are: pre-frontal cortex, the pre-motor area and the motor area.

The clusters of neurons included in the *prefrontal cortex* have at least nine important functions, each of which is involved in an individual's quest to become master of body, mind and emotions. These are:

a) Regulation of the body
Balance is required between the two parts of the autonomic nervous system: the sympathetic nervous system (the SNS: that which ensures our physical survival through the fight/flight/freeze/faint mechanism) and the parasympathetic nervous system (the PNS: that which lulls the body into inactivity, repose and rest). When the two are out of balance, either the Human Value of Peace remains inaccessible (overactive SNS) or Right Conduct is inhibited (overactive PNS).

b) Attuned communication – felt sense of other's experience

The Human Value of Truth can be seen as being active here in that – there being no two, only the Oneness – those who are sharing (relating) their experiences with each other are going beyond the physical and mental constructs of separateness to have a sense of identification with the other, as if there were only the Oneness.

c) Regulation of emotions

Those who have the ability to notice, make room for (within themselves), and then regulate their emotions are better able to clear the road for their innate Human Values to emerge. Anger, fear and envy keep us away from pure Love; agitation, impatience and boredom banish our Peace; argumentativeness, pride and self-pity leave no room for us to experience Truth; greed, sloth and selfishness stand in the way of Right Conduct; while unforgiveness, jealousy and hatred preclude us from practising Non-violence.

d) Response flexibility – pause, options, evaluate options, appropriate decision

This function of the pre-frontal cortex underlies the adages of 'think before you speak' and 'count to ten before you react'. It allows time and space for one's commitment to a virtuous life to rise up and be given the opportunity to manifest itself. When we pause, we are, in effect, like the regal passenger (the higher Self) in the horse-drawn coach (the body) saying to the driver (the conscience) who sits up top, "Use the reins (the mind) to bring the horses (the emotions and the senses) under control so that we can pause for a while and see where is the best direction to go." The Human Values of Truth and Peace, in particular, are activated here when we stand back from (not identify with) the body, mind and emotions.

e) Empathy

The philosophy embracing the five Human Values principle says that empathy, compassion and altruism are innate human qualities but, like the burning coals that get covered with the ash of the fire, these inborn virtues can fall below conscious awareness until fanned into a blaze by an inspiring mentor or awakening experience. We are hard-wired to feel another's pain and joy because, according to both quantum physics and universal spirituality, we are not separate, any more than one wave in the vast ocean is separate from another. To understand and accept this means embracing the Human Values of Truth and Love.

To be empathic is to breathe the air of Love; it is to convey to the afflicted, without any words being spoken, that our Love impels us to feel their pain as much as we are open to it. To be able to feel the full extent of another's emotions is only possible when we know from our own experience that we are the Witness of these emotions, not the emotions themselves. When we can feel the pain underlying another's anger directed towards us, we are practising Non-violence which is, as you know, infused with Love.

f) Insight – self-awareness

The faculty of insight allows us to see ourselves as others see us; to shine a light on our own shadows and blindspots; and to discover an underlying truth or pattern that makes sense of the chaos or confusion. When an impasse in problem solving is reached using logical reasoning, a certain relaxation or letting-go allows the pre-frontal cortex to shift the search from within the left hemisphere (reason) to the right hemisphere (no reason). That is how insight occurs. Insight is possible to the extent that we have an open mind, by-passing logical thinking and fixed ideas, sufficient to allow one to taste a drop from the vast, limitless ocean of Truth where all knowledge resides.

g) Fear extinction – GABA fibres to amygdala

The limbic region of the brain is the seat of our emotional learning and the amygdala is its most well-known structure, generating the 'fight or flight' response when it is triggered by the sympathetic nervous system. To ensure that we do not react our way into fear-driven isolationism, neuronal axons (fibres) generated by the pre-frontal cortex carry GABA (gamma butyric acid) down to the amygdala to extinguish the fear response. The Human Values philosophy recognises that the fires of Peace, Love and Non-violence are kindled when we nurture the growth of the pre-frontal cortex to refine its regulating role.

h) Intuition – deep knowing without logic

Our 'sixth sense' is one of the paths for awakening to the Human Value of Truth. With aspects in common with insight, intuition leaps ahead of the logical mind to sense what is yet to be revealed – perhaps future events, or following our 'path that has heart'. It is as if we fly to the stars on the wings of intuition, then build the ladder of logic and reason so that our rational mind can follow. It is only when there is a willingness to let go of fixed ideas or plans, wants and disappointments – when the mind is open and still – that intuition speaks loud and clear. The pre-frontal cortex facilitates this necessary shift in allegiance from the left side of the brain to the right, from whence intuition arises.

i) Morality – behaviours based on empathy

With the understanding that all of creation is interconnected in a holographic manner – 'I am in you, and you are in me' – it is our ability to feel another's joy and sorrow that prompts us to behave in ways that enhance the happiness of others and relieve their pain, or at least to cause no pain. Empathy is a facet of the Human Value of Love, and morality arises out of, and is expressed as Love. Morality is described by the five Human Values of Love, Peace, Truth, Right Conduct and Non-violence, each one of which is a pure steam flowing out of the one eternal spring of Love.

- Mirror neurons – as the name suggests – have been identified as being responsible for imitation learning or vicarious conditioning. Their presence in the brain partly explains how children learn basic skills like speaking a language, opening a door, behaving socially, expressing emotions and, in all likelihood, developing character traits.

  What happens is that, when we observe somebody behaving in a particular way, our mirror neurons begin setting up patterns of reactivity that ensure we will mirror, mimic or imitate what our senses are taking in. Of particular interest for our cause is that our mirror neurons fire off in increasing numbers according to the emotional intensity or passion of the one we are observing. We see it in rioting, football team chanting, whole continents reacting with fear to a new disease pandemic, and perhaps even an image going viral on the internet.

  If mirror neurons are playing such a major role in the sudden coming together of many minds along a common theme, it is likely that the same neurological triggers are in play when we are inspired by some noble personalities to aim for human excellence. Knowing this, we are given even more incentive to find within ourselves the Love of a Mother Teresa, the Peace of a St. Francis of Assisi, the Truth of an Abraham Lincoln, the Right Conduct of a Florence Nightingale and the Non-violence of a Mahatma Gandhi.

  If we can commit ourselves to living the five Human Values with humility, passion and earnestness, we can assume that others who care about or look up to us will, through the activity of their mirror neurons, automatically create the conditions within themselves for a virtuous character to emerge and flourish.

Defining the Mind

The neuropsychiatrist Dan Siegel in his 2007 book, *The Mindful Brain: Reflection and Attunement in the Cultivation of Well-Being*, suggests that, if all relevant researchers – from anthropologists to neuroscientists – could find a common language for describing the mind it would be:

> *The mind is an embodied and relational process that regulates the flow of energy and information as it is shared within relationships, and as it moves through the mechanisms of the brain, and the neural connections within the nervous system distributed through the whole body.*

While the above definition is important for the exacting language of science, a more simple and useful explanation of the mind is given by Sathya Sai Baba:

> *The mind is nothing but a bundle of desires. If you separate threads, cloth disappears. Similarly, if you remove desires, one by one, the mind ceases to exist. It is the mind that makes a man or mars him. If it is immersed in things of the world, it leads to bondage; if it treats the world as but temporary, then by that discipline it becomes free and light.*

As Dan Siegel has pointed out, all modern researchers in the mind/brain/relationship fields agree that the mind has very powerful functions, directing the physiological and neurological aspects of the body in a highly complex way - what we think, determines our physical, social, emotional and mental health. Siegel (2007) also says:

> *The mind is not an entity – it is an ongoing process that organises itself. On the one hand it is arising from the interaction between the energy/information flowing within the body and that which is*

shared between people. On the other hand it is also providing feedback that regulates these very flows of energy/information out of which it is arising. This means that our relationships and our brains shape our mind, and our mind shapes our relationships and our brain.

The teachings of Buddhism tell us that all of our suffering comes from wanting things of this world. Since the mind is made up of desires, we can replace worldly cravings with the more noble, selfless and elevating desires such as the wish to be kind and have compassion, to be forgiving and non-judgmental, to be courageous and calm.

As we can see from the above synopsis of modern mind/brain/relationship research, the mind has enormous potential for taking our ship of state either onto the rocks or out to the freedom of the open sea. Further, our social and physical environment – what comes into us through the five senses – can change the function and structure of our brain, which in turn influences how we think and what we do. Therefore, the more often we think and act in a virtuous way, the more will our brains be restructured so as to facilitate this more noble way of thinking and behaving.

Brain, Emotions and Learning

With the development of new methods for studying the functions of different parts of the brain, there is now consensus that emotions involve the body, brain and the mind. Specific brain systems manifest the emotions in the body (e.g. breathing, temperature, etc.), in sensations (physical pain and pleasure, etc.), and in changing thought content (e.g. thoughts of revenge when angered, altruistic ideas when loving and compassionate, etc.). In each case the emotion can be played out on the face and in the body, or it can sometimes involve representations of bodily sensations that do not leave the brain. Reflecting on these findings and others, neuroscientists and educationists Mary Helen Immordino-Yang and Antonio Damasio write in their 2007 publication, *We Feel, Therefore We Learn:*

> *And in each case, these feelings interact with other thoughts to change the mind in characteristic ways, and to help people learn from their experiences. Put simply, what affective neuroscience is revealing is that the mind is influenced by an interdependency of the body and brain; both the body and brain are involved, therefore, in learning.*

We also know from neuroscience that the emotional and cognitive functions are not discrete structures in the brain. Certainly the limbic system – particularly the amygdala – plays a major role in the emotions, and the hippocampus and pre-frontal cortex likewise for cognition. However, the pre-frontal cortex (PFC) and amygdala are linked and have strong connections between them so that each can influence the other. For emotional regulation, the PFC (our social brain) exerts influence over the rapid emotional signalling and response of the amygdala, while the latter can link with the PFC to drive enthusiasm, motivation, and socialisation (which includes attachment). Linda Graham, in her 2008 paper, *The Neuroscience of Attachment,* wrote:

> *John Bowlby, British psychoanalyst, founder of attachment theory, hypothesized that attachment is all about safety and protection and emotional regulation in times of perceived threat or danger. Attachment is part of a 3-part motivational system of fear-attachment-exploration. Fear triggers attachment behaviours. The safe haven of secure attachment soothes the fear of the amygdala, and opens exploration ... Exploration eventually bumps us into something that triggers fear*

again which shuts down exploration and triggers attachment behaviours again which soothe the fear again and opens the exploration cycle of safety-exploration again ...

Those who did not feel cared for and understood in their early years of childhood carry with them the emotional scars of anxiety, depression, anger, distrust of relationships, self-doubt and social immaturity. Such people, in particular, are ever in search of an antidote for their inner pain. So it is important for them to find and spend time with adult role models who are exemplars of Love, Peace, Truth, Right Conduct and Non-violence. Through the medium of their mirror neurons, every experience in the company of such people will help to build positive neural networks in their own brain (particularly in the right hemisphere) that will progressively balance out and neutralize the negative ones. With such changes taking place in the brain structure, and thereby functioning, they will feel increasingly motivated to rediscover the very best within themselves.

In her pioneering neuroscientific and clinical work, Linda Graham has explained how utilising tools that appeal to the right hemisphere of the brain (the holistic, non-logical, non-linguistic side) can undo negative imprints from our childhood.

There are some effective methods developed by psychologists that can be used by anyone who has persistent emotional difficulties whose genesis may have been in early childhood. These exercises all create an imaginary mother or father figure who is consistently loving and non-judgmental, or a Wise Being who accompanies us through dfficult situations.

As noted earlier, the philosophy underlying the Human Values approach regards all emotions as waves of energy with the potential to carry us to a higher level of one or more of the Values, towards Peaceful Mind and Open Heart. If the emotion is positive we can use our thoughts and imagination to increase or expand the joy, gratitude, love, enthusiasm and so on. If the emotion is a negative one, we can look inwardly, using our intuition or insight, to find a feeling that transmutes the negative into the positive. For example, the feelings of grief can be transmuted into profound and delicate feelings of gentleness; feelings of envy or avarice can change into compassion when we think of people who have little or nothing (poor, starving, in prison and so on), or animals that are being neglected or cruelly treated.

The image to illustrate this transformational process is that of the stretched bow shooting an arrow towards a target. The emotion is the tension in the bow. The arrow is our mind. The target is Peaceful Mind and Open Heart. If the arrow (the mind) is pointed away from the target, we do not get to experience the joy, the peace, the love, the grandeur that we are. If the emotion (the tension in the bow) is restricted or shut away from our awareness, there is insufficient power for the arrow to reach the target, even if it is accurately pointed in the right direction. That is, when we allow ourselves to feel an emotion fully (whether joy, adulation, loneliness or anger), and turn the mind towards the ideal – the Treasure both within and all around – the emotion releases the positive neurotransmitters in the brain to jump across the millions of synapses in the neural circuits that promote human excellence.

As noted earlier, it is clear that everything existing in Nature is exquisitely arranged in perfect order so as to give us the perfection that supports and surrounds us. We are part of Nature, and so it follows that every emotion has its role to play in guiding us towards experiencing the human excellence (Peaceful Mind, Open Heart) that we always have been.

We are like Kings and Queens who are asleep, and our emotions are wake-up calls for us to arise and reclaim our regal heritage, the priceless Treasure that we all are. And our brains and minds are exquisitely designed, in concert with our heart, body and nervous system, to take us on this Royal Road to awakening.

Being with whatever arises,
working with the tendencies of mind to transform them,
and taking refuge in the ground of Being
are the essential practices
of the path of awakening.

Rick Hanson

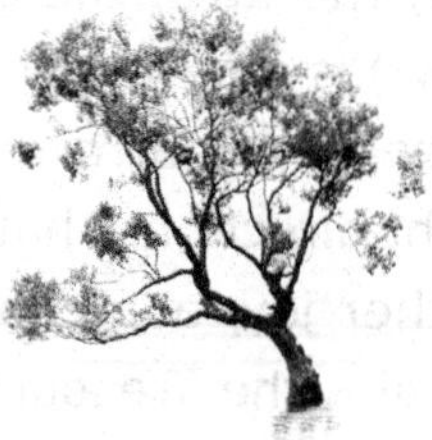

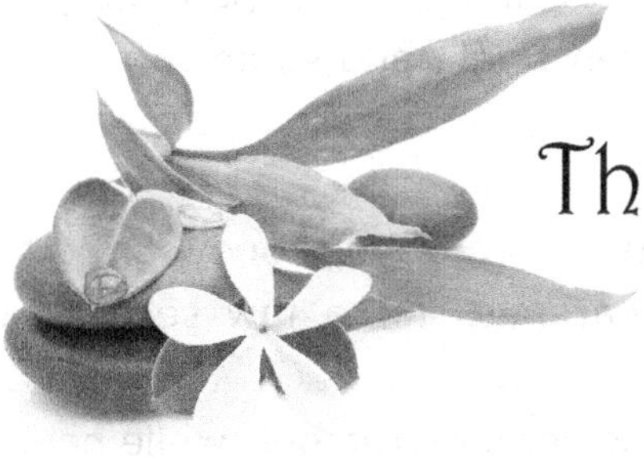

The Practice

EXERCISES TO REGULATE THE MIND AND THE BRAIN

Exercise 1:

Engaging the Parasympathetic Nervous System - Relaxation

How can I do this exercise?

◇ Brief relaxation
  - Relax your eyes, tongue and jaw muscles.
  - Run warm water over your hands.
  - Scan your body for areas that are tense, and relax them as well as you can.
  - Imagine (feel) tension draining out of your body down into the earth.

◇ Diaphragm breathing
  - Place your open palms over the stomach (diaphragm) so that you can see how much you can extend it while inhaling.
  - Breath like a baby, pushing the stomach out as you breathe in.
  - Do this for 10 breaths only, once every day if you can, until this is your natural way of breathing.

◇ Progressive relaxation
  - For a few minutes, focus progressively on different parts of the body.

- Focus for 5 seconds on small units of the body (left foot, left ankle, left calf muscle, left knee, left thigh, and so on).

◇ Spot relaxation
- When you become aware of a tense area of your body, bring the various sensations there into awareness for a few seconds or longer.
- Say 'relax' softly or in your mind as you breathe out, while having that awareness of the body part (e.g. left shoulder).

Exercise 2:
Heart Focus

How can I do this exercise?

◇ Focus on your breath, counting silently so that inhalation and exhalation are of the same duration (e.g. 4 seconds each).
◇ While doing this, imagine the breath going directly into and out of your heart. Place a hand (or both hands) over the chest.
◇ As you breathe evenly through your heart, see if you can remember the most joyful, contented, happy or loving experience you've ever had. Imagine this feeling move through your heart as part of the breath.

Exercise 3:
Big Exhalation

How can I do this exercise?
◇ Inhale as much as you can and hold it for a few seconds; then exhale slowly while relaxing. This activates the parasympathetic ner-

vous system, which is in charge of exhaling. Do this 3 or 4 times to begin with.

◇ With practice, you can increase the effect of this by inhaling, holding and exhaling according to a time ratio of 2, 8 and 4. For example, you might count 4 seconds to inhale deeply, hold that for 16 seconds, and take 8 seconds to exhale.

Let your mind wander in the pure and simple.
Be one with the infinite.
Let all things take their course.

Chuang Tsu

Chapter 7

The Heart-Brain Connection

May you experience each day as a sacred gift
woven around the heart of wonder.

John O'Donohue

While many cultural and spiritual traditions throughout history have shared a regard for the heart as a source of wisdom and positive emotions such as love, care, appreciation and compassion, recent scientific discoveries suggest that these long-surviving associations may indeed be more than merely metaphorical. In particular, new understandings of the physiology of positive emotions and the key role played by the heart in the generation of emotional experience have positive implications for education, physical and mental health, authentic happiness, psychosocial wellbeing and awakening to our innate Peaceful Mind , Open Heart.

It was Aristotle in early Greece who argued for a heart-centred model of learning, memory and intelligence, one that proposed that the heart is the organ of intelligence. This cardiocentric view supplanted the brain-centred (encephalocentric) model of Plato, his teacher, and survived well into the 16th century when Galen (the father of experimental psychology) demonstrated the vital role of the brain. Since that time there has been a tremendous amount of research carried out investigating the functions and structure of the brain.

While most neurophysiological research has been focussed on the brain, a few significant studies, beginning in the 1960's, have examined the neural 'conversations' between the heart and brain. In particular, the pioneer physiologists John and Beatrice Lacey observed that the heart actually communicates with the brain, and that input from the heart and cardiovascular system could significantly influence both perception and behaviour (sensory-motor integration). Since that time, attention has shifted more to how signals from the heart to the brain affect our ability to think clearly, focus attention, recall information, learn and reason. The nature of this input coming from the heart is determined by the positivity or negativity of our emotions.

Emotions and the Heart's Rhythms

Many of the recent investigations into the heart-brain connection have been carried out by the Institute of HeartMath in the USA. These researchers have identified heart rate variability (HRV) as being a promising tool in examining the interactions between the heart and brain. The term HRV describes those naturally-occurring, beat-to-beat changes in heart rate. Recent research has shown that heart rate variability patterns are directly influenced by changes in emotional states.

What seems to happen is that, when we are caught up in negative emotions (such as anxiety, sadness, frustration and anger), the two branches of our autonomic nervous system stop moderating, or synchronising with, each other. The sympathetic nervous system arouses us to 'fight or flight' while the parasympathetic nervous system is calming us down. There is an ideal balance between these two nervous systems for optimum physiological and cognitive functioning, and this happens when we have sustained, positive emotions such as kindness, compassion, love and gratitude. At such times our patterns of heart rhythm are highly ordered or *coherent.*

The terms *cardiac coherence* and *physiological coherence* are used interchangeably in the research literature, and need some explaining. When one inhales, one's heart rate increases, and it decreases when one exhales, which leads to a physiological variation of the time between two heart beats – referred to as heart rate variability or HRV.

Sustained, heart-felt, positive emotions result in an ordered, symmetric HRV. When HRV is symmetric (that is when there is a sine wave-like pattern in the time between heart beats), the autonomic nervous system (ANS) is perfectly balanced and harmonious; but when it isn't symmetric it is a sign that the ANS, in particular, has been activated to respond to stress. The state of perfect symmetry in HRV can be described as cardiac coherence which helps our brain and body to function better intellectually, emotionally, socially and physically. When we are stressed and our emotions are negative, our heart rhythms become more chaotic and disorganised (less coherent), which interferes with all of our brain and bodily functions.

The Heart-Brain Connection and Human Values

As noted earlier, an important part of the Human Values philosophy is the dictum that each one of the five Human Values of Love, Truth, Peace, Right Conduct and Non-violence already lies within every human being, in full measure, largely hidden from conscious awareness but manifested in so many acts of kindness, courage, altruism and honesty in our everyday life. As one striking example of this, psychologists have observed that almost all children aged between 14 and 18 months will spontaneously pick up a clothes peg and hand it to an experimenter who had 'accidentally' dropped it and was 'struggling' to pick it up, this without any encouragement, and within 5 seconds. However the children will make no attempt to engage in this altruistic behaviour if the person drops the object 'intentionally'.

During these experiments, the adult never asks for help verbally, and most of the time does not even look in the direction of the child to indicate that he has trouble picking up the clothes peg. The child will help each time the clothes peg is dropped. However, if praise or a reward is given, the altruistic behaviour drops off quickly. This appears to indicate that the child is motivated to help for purely unselfish reasons. Felix Warneken, one of the authors of the 2009 research paper, *The Roots of Altruism*, notes:

> *The results were astonishing because these children are so young – they still wear diapers and are barely able to use language, but they already show helping behaviour.*

These findings are but one of many reported by Matthieu Ricard in his 2013 book, *Altruism: The Power of Compassion to Change Yourself and the World*, indicating that all of the Human Values are intrinsically present at a very early age. This innate moral sense begins to be attenuated as the child grows older, with sharing and helping and other behaviours becoming less universal in their expression, depending upon the moral character of parents and teachers.

The abundance of psychological research into the compassionate and altruistic behaviour of very young children suggests that the heart, relatively free as yet from any qualifying cognitive feedback from the brain, is the main organ – rather than the brain – that is instrumental in instigating humane and moral behaviour. This is our common experience when we look into the eyes and face of a baby - whose presence can soon attract a crowd of strangers to interact with it more so than any adult ever could. What we see is the essence of 'no-mind' looking unblinkingly back at us; only purity and authenticity are there.

As we've said earlier, the Human Value of Love – pure, lasting, unconditional, selfless, ever-expanding and inclusive Love – is the foundation principle, the essence, underlying each one of the other four Human Values of Truth, Peace, Right Conduct and Non-violence. Without Love, there can be no real peace; nor will our actions be righteous and non-violent, with only a distorted form of Truth being present. As Sathya Sai Baba says:

> *The values a man must cherish as his life-breath are: Truth, Righteousness, Peace, Love and Non-violence. Of these five vital principles, Love is the foremost. It is Love that flows as the under-current for the other four Values. How does it flow this way? When Love is associated with our thoughts, it manifests itself as Truth. When Love is associated with feelings, it produces Peace. When Love animates actions, it results in Right Action. When Love is combined with understanding, it becomes Non-violence. Therefore, whenever you feel angry, think of Love, develop thoughts of Love in your heart. You will have Peace.*

These words accord with the spiritual teachings of all faiths and creeds, the essence of which points to the heart as the place in the body from which all goodness derives, with the role of the mind being to ensure that all paths remain open to the guidance and influence from this Holy Grail. It is a two-way process, with the mind being guided by an open heart, and the heart being nurtured into its true flowering by a mind soaked in wisdom. The heart is akin to a light bulb which can only glow with Love when the current flowing into it is from a mind that sees only the oneness of humanity (Truth) – that is, seeing ourself in all, and so loving everyone the same. When Love is shared, Peace reigns – Peaceful Mind, Open Heart.

If we were to assign a personality to the heart organ we would say that it is soaked in Love, motivated by Love, because all of its activities are in the selfless service of every other neuron, cell, bone, tissue and organ in the body. If the heart ceases to do its work, the body becomes lifeless. Further, the heart is the first organ to form during development of the body in the womb, with the first heart beats occurring just four weeks after conception. Its role is immediately and totally one of service, pumping blood through the circulatory system to carry nutrients to, and waste away from, the surrounding cells in the developing embryo. Its whole life and purpose is one of loving, selfless service to the entire body.

Even before the heart begins to form, from the moment of conception the whole process of cell formation can be seen as Love in action. In his 1974 book of essays, *The Lives of a Cell,* immunology researcher Lewis Thomas reasons that life on earth has evolved through cooperation between the various elements of Nature. He compares the Earth to a living cell, one with its own membrane (the atmosphere) that is the 'grandest product of collaboration in all of Nature'. The whole process of evolution would seem to be Love in action. If so, then life is Love.

The role of the heart in the human body is that every day it pumps over 100,000 times, sending blood to the lungs where it gets purified on its way to nurture all parts of the body. Each time the heart beats, the pumped blood begins its journey of 32,000 kilometres throughout the body. Again we can see that it lives a life totally in the service of the rest of the body – Love in action.

We know from research studies that the heart sends information to the brain, influencing cognition and sensory input (e.g. We do not see so well when the heart rate variability becomes disordered because of a negative emotion, and our learning and recall are diminished also). Recent studies indicate that the heart also communicates through its electromagnetic field. The electrical component of the heart's field is 60 times stronger than that of the brain's, and permeates every cell in the body. The magnetic component of the heart's field is approximately 5000 times stronger than the brain's, and can be detected several metres away from the body using sensitive equipment.

At the Institute of HeartMath, Rollin McCraty and others have found early evidence that the heart's electromagnetic field can transmit information between people who are almost two metres apart. In fact, the brain of a person is able to synchronise itself with the electromagnetic field of another person's heart who is nearby. This suggests that one of the mechanisms for empathy and social connectedness between people could be the heart's electromagnetic field. Not surprisingly, the future could see a clear scientific explanation of aspects of the Human Value of Love becoming available.

Another striking finding is that the heart and brain can both detect an event before it has happened, with the heart receiving this intuitive information earlier than the brain. This intriguing finding opens possibilities for future research that could identify the electromagnetic field of the heart as a mechanism for intuitive perception. Intuition is seen as one of the aspects of the Human Value of Truth.

These early studies into the heart suggest that it is much more than a pump that circulates blood. Although it has only 40,000 neurons compared to the brain's 100 billion or so, the heart appears to have its own functioning brain. The new discipline of neurocardiology shows that the heart is not only a sensory organ (as indicated above) but also has a nervous system (the 'heart brain') that enables it to learn, remember, and make functional decisions independent of the brain's cerebral cortex. It is feasible that, through the signals that the heart is continuously sending to the higher brain centres involved in perception, cognition, emotional processing and physiological balance, the heart could be playing a guiding role in our awakening to our innate Human Values, to our inborn human excellence.

Overall, the research in the fields of neurocardiology, psychophysiology, and neuroscience together support the idea that the heart could have an inherent intelligence and wisdom worth being 'listened' to and acted upon. In a 2012 article (see: www.heartmath.org), titled *Heart Intelligence*, the Institute of HeartMath wrote:

> *Heart intelligence is the flow of awareness, understanding and intuition we experience when the mind and emotions are brought into coherent alignment with the heart. It can be activated through self-initiated practice, and the more we pay attention when we sense the heart is speaking to us or guiding us, the greater our ability to access this intelligence and guidance more frequently.*
>
> *Heart intelligence actually transfers intelligence to the emotions and instils the power of emotional management. In other words, heart intelligence is really the source of emotional intelligence ... It is through learning how to decipher messages we receive from our heart that we gain the keen perception needed to effectively manage our emotions in the midst of life's challenges.*

Because a high level of cardiac coherence appears to be the ideal condition for the heart's intelligence to perform its guiding, balancing functions most effectively, and because the presence or self-induction of positive feelings can help facilitate this, we have the opportunity to influence profoundly our destiny in a positive way, perhaps utilising some of the exercises to follow.

The utterances of the Heart
- unlike those of the discriminating intellect -
always relate to the whole.

Carl Gustav Jung

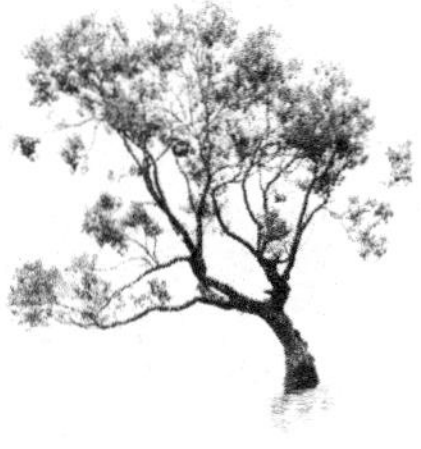

The Practice

EXERCISES FOR CULTIVATING HEART INTELLIGENCE
(CARDIAC COHERENCE)

The ability to alter our emotional responses is central to our overall well-being, and can help us on our journey along the path of awakening to our inborn human excellence. There is a feedback loop between our emotions and the availability of our heart's intelligence. Let us explore a number of well-tested techniques for self-inducing positive emotions so as to establish optimal cardiac coherence.

<u>Exercise 1:</u>

Cardiac Coherence: Heart-focussed Breathing

How can I do this exercise?

◇ Focus your attention in the area of your heart.

◇ Imagine your breath is flowing in and out of your heart or chest area, breathing a little slower and deeper than usual. You could take 5 seconds to inhale, and 5 seconds to exhale, or whatever feels comfortable for you.

◇ Use your imagination to experience a positive, regenerative feeling such as being calm or having gratitude or loving-care for someone or something in your life. You might like to re-experience a special feeling you have for someone you love, or for a pet, a special place, or something you have achieved, etc.

◇ Do this for 5 to 10 minutes, 2 or 3 times every day.

<u>Exercise 2:</u>

Cardiac Coherence: Self-Induced Positive Feeling

How can I do this exercise?

◇ Without any attempt to regulate your breathing, decide to self-activate a positive or calming feeling. You might like to try self-inducing any one of the following emotions: kindness, friendliness, caring, compassion, calmness, serenity, gratitude, courage, happiness, awe, exultation, patience, equanimity, forgiveness, acceptance, serenity, confidence, love, or feeling loved.

◇ Sometimes it helps to allow the feeling to take you back in time to an occasion that may have lasted for a minute or a month, when that feeling was very strong.

◇ Use your imagination to magnify, expand and multiply that feeling.

◇ Now imagine that the feeling is in every cell in your body.

◇ Place your hand over the centre of your chest (touch opens the heart still further).

◇ Imagine that every breath brings more of that feeling into you.

◇ Imagine that the feeling is all around you, above and below you, in front of you and behind you, to the right and left of you, going all the way to infinity.

◇ Do this for 10 to 15 minutes, twice every day.

<u>Exercise 3:</u>
Cardiac Coherence: Heart Lock-In

How can I do this exercise?

◇ In this exercise the aim is to spend a longer time focussing on a loving feeling in the heart. It is spending time nourishing the garden of your heart.

◇ Find a quiet place, close your eyes and relax. Focussing your attention on your heart, pretend that you are breathing slowly through it. Do this for 20 to 30 seconds.

◇ Remember the feeling of love or care for someone whom it is easy for you to love. Or you can focus on a feeling of appreciation for someone or something positive in your life. Try to stay with that feeling for between 5 and 15 minutes, quite a long time.

◇ When thoughts take you away, gently let go of them, and bring your focus back to your heart. If the energy feels too intense or your heart feels blocked or tight, let go of any tension in the body and imagine you can feel a softness all through your heart.

◇ Gently send that feeling of love, care or appreciation to yourself.

◇ Now send that feeling to others, one by one, then more and more, until you are radiating it to the whole world.

Exercise 4:

Cardiac Coherence: The Tree of Love

How can I do this exercise?

◇ Make yourself comfortable. Close your eyes to practise each step, and then open them to read the next.

◇ This is a journey of imagination. Imagine that you see a very special tree. You walk right up to it and stand with your back to the trunk. Imagine that you feel one with this tree. You are the tree. Do this for 10 to 15 seconds.

◇ As you breathe in, imagine that a perfect fatherly love – the love of a thousand ideal fathers – is flowing down into your branches from above. Do this for 5 breaths.

◇ Now, as your breathe in, imagine that a perfect motherly love – the love of a thousand ideal mothers – is flowing up into you through your roots. Do this for 5 breaths.

◇ Now imagine that perfect fatherly love and the perfect motherly love are pouring into you each time you breathe in, flowing down into you from above, and up from below, filling you up. Do this for 5 to 10 breaths.

◇ Now imagine that both of these loves keep pouring into you, independent of the breath, filling you up, and that Love is now radiating out from every pore in your skin, shining out to the whole world. Do this for as long as you like, once every day for a while.

The best and most beautiful things in the world
cannot be seen or even touched.
They must be felt with the heart.

Helen Keller

Part Three

Embracing the Path of Aging

I am larger, better than I thought,
I did not know I held so
much goodness.

Walt Whitman

Chapter 8

Health and Wellbeing in Old Age

For age is opportunity no less
than youth itself, though in another dress,
and as the evening twilight fades away
the sky is filled with stars invisible by day.

Henry Wadsworth Longfellow

The human body has evolved over the eons to become a highly-advanced, biological machine that appears to have infinite potential. As with all machines, human aging brings with it a general slowing down and the need for some repairs and support with advancing years. Generally, machines that have been respected and cared for throughout their lives require less maintenance in their closing years. This is a message that could strike a chord with many of us. That is, to the extent that we can learn to regulate our emotions, master our thoughts, be physically healthy and dive deep within ourselves to connect with our Peaceful Mind and Open Heart throughout the different stages of our life, this extraordinary machine in which we reside for perhaps 60 to 100 years is more likely to serve us well in our later years.

Life is a journey and, if there is a desert to cross before we reach our destination, it would be wise to prepare for that part of the journey – where the pace is slower and the demands greater – while we are still travelling through the lush countryside. The old adage, 'A stitch in time saves nine', is appropriate here. For example, if we have not developed the habit of feeling grateful several times every day during our more 'lush' years, it will be very difficult to even notice the beauty of the desert flowers, the awesome power of the all-consuming silence, and to know where to look for those hidden reservoirs of water when finally we are traversing across the markedly different landscape of our later years.

Such preparation for the closing years was not so necessary until the early 1900's. The 20th century, during which most of us were born, witnessed two profound changes in those regions of the world where people are well educated and science and technology flourish. Life expectancy nearly doubled and fertility rates fell dramatically. As a result, individuals and whole populations are aging. It is only recently that we have realised the importance of conducting research into these later 30 to 50 years of life that have been added on to the first 40 or so. Much of this chapter examines some of the more relevant aspects of research that relates to the underlying theme of much of this book: the quest for a lasting happiness that will endure and be accessible during our closing years.

Psychological Health and Wellbeing in Old Age

Psychological wellbeing and health are closely related, and the link may become more important at older ages, if only because the prevalence of chronic illness generally increases with advancing years. Studies of older people indicate that quality of life is affected by a person's state of health, but the unexpected finding that life satisfaction mostly increases with age suggests that psychological wellbeing is affected by many factors other than health.

Impaired psychological wellbeing is often a precursor to increased risk of physical illness. There is an established research literature linking depression and life stress with premature mortality, coronary heart disease, diabetes, disability and other chronic conditions. It is generally agreed that psychological wellbeing may even be a protective factor in health, reducing the risk of chronic physical illness and promoting longevity.

Among lifestyle factors, physical activity is probably the most important link between psychological wellbeing and health. Regular physical activity at older ages is already recommended for the maintenance of cardiovascular health, muscle strength and flexibility, glucose metabolism, and healthy body weight, and is also consistently correlated with wellbeing.

Psychological Capacities in Old Age

Changes in the psychological capacities of individuals over the adult lifespan have been well studied. So that we can gain a better understanding of how a decline in physical and mental functioning can have an impact on our general happiness and life satisfaction, let's explore in detail what we now know about some of the different aspects of aging.

Sensory function

The changes in the central nervous system and in the peripheral sensory receptors and their specialized structures result in reduced sensory input with age. Thus, an older person generally does not hear and see so well. Another effect of the reduced sensory input may be the lowering of the total level of excitation imparted to the neurons, thereby affecting the level of activity of the individual.

Speed and timing

One of the most distinguishing features of aging persons is their tendency to behave lethargically. Whereas young adults behave quickly or slowly in accord with the demands of the situation, older adults generally move at a slower rate, independent of the situation.

The overall slowness of behaviour in older persons is looked upon as being most probably due to general aging of the nervous system and neuronal systems in the brain. Explanations involve the loss of nerve cells, reduced neural excitability, physical-chemical changes at the synapse that limit transmission speed, and a lowered excitation resulting from changes in subcortical centres.

Cognitive Functions

Much of what follows in this section on mental proficiency in the aged has been guided by material in the chapter by Elizabeth Glisky, *Changes in Cognitive Function in Human Aging*, in the 2007 book edited by David Riddle, *Brain Aging: Models, Methods, Mechanisms.*

As people age, they change in many ways, both biological and psychological. Some of these changes can be for the better, and others are not. Disease, particularly cerebrovascular and primary brain disease in late life, can seriously impair mental functioning and limit effective behaviour.

There is ample evidence that alterations in brain structure and functions are intimately tied to alterations in cognitive function, and the relationship between the two can often change at various times across the lifespan. In this section we will explore changes in cognitive functioning, with the understanding that many of these will be related to some form of deterioration in the brain.

Basic cognitive functions

◇ Attention

Older adults show significant impairments on attentional tasks that require the dividing or switching of attention among multiple inputs or tasks. They show relative preservation of performance on tasks that require selection of relevant stimuli; and, although they are slower than young adults, they are not necessarily distracted more. Also they are able to maintain concentration for an extended period of time. The tasks on which older adults show impairment tend to be those that require flexible control of attention, a cognitive function associated with the frontal lobes. Importantly, these types of tasks appear to be amenable to training and can benefit from improved cardiovascular fitness. If the attentional deficits are severe this can have a significant impact on an older person's ability to function adequately and independently in everyday life.

◇ Working memory

Older adults tend to do poorly on tasks that involve active manipulation, reorganization, or integration of the contents of working memory.

A decline in working memory can make life quite difficult for an elderly person because many complex everyday tasks such as decision-making, problem-solving, and the planning of goal-directed behaviours require the integration and reorganization of information from a variety of sources. It seems likely that attention, speed of information processing, and the ability to inhibit irrelevant information are all important functions for effective performance of these higher-level cognitive tasks.

◇ Long-term memory

Aging principally affects episodic memory, namely, memory for specific events or experiences that occurred in the past. Although many older adults believe that their memories for remote events are better than their memories for recent events, it is likely that older memories have become more semantic or gist-like, retaining the general core information but lacking details, particularly where and when the event took place. More problematic for older adults is remembering whether something actually happened or was just thought about.

◇ Perception

Declining sensory and perceptual abilities have important implications for the everyday lives of older adults. Hearing loss can isolate older people, preventing them from engaging in conversation and other social interactions. Visual impairments can limit mobility and interact with attentional deficits to make driving a particularly hazardous activity. As older people develop strategies to compensate for declining sensory abilities, the ways in which they perform other cognitive tasks may also be altered and may become less efficient.

Higher-level cognitive functions

◇ Speech and language

Speech and language processing are largely intact in older adults under normal conditions, although their processing time may be somewhat slower than in young adults. In fact, there is evidence that conversation skills actually improve with age. Older people often tell well-structured elaborate narratives that are judged by others to be more interesting than those told by younger adults.

◇ Decision making

Most of the research work in the field of aging has highlighted the potential impact of attentional and working memory limitations on the ability to make decisions, but it has also indicated that factors such as motivation, relevance, emotional investment, and prior knowledge can be important moderators of those effects, particularly in real-life contexts. Research has shown that, when making decisions in real-life situations, older adults often arrive at the same kinds of outcomes as younger adults but reach their conclusions in a different way. They tend to rely more on prior knowledge about the problem domain and less on new information.

◇ Executive control

As noted in earlier chapters, the pre-frontal cortex (PFC) at the front of the brain is responsible for a complex array of mental skills.

In addition to what we learned about the role of the pre-frontal cortex in helping us to develop good character, neuroscientists have also established that it is responsible for a complex array of mental skills for helping us to get things done – psychologists refer to these cognitive abilities as *executive function*. These executive control functions include the abilities to: differentiate among competing thoughts; determine what is good and bad, better and best, same and different; ascertain the future consequences of present activities; work towards a defined goal; make predictions of outcomes; and suppress urges that, if not subdued, could lead to socially-unacceptable outcomes.

Studies using neuroimaging show that, as we move into later elder years, there is a steady decline in both the volume and ability of the PFC brain region. That is, our executive control could weaken as we age, which can make life increasingly challenging. However, there are a number of steps that can be taken to compensate for any such decline, some of which are included as exercises in The Practice at the end of this chapter.

Wellbeing in Old Age

Older people are often thought of as being lonely, hopeless and sad. The general belief is that, because cognitive and physical decline usually accompanies aging, so too will happiness and life satisfaction become less. One of the leading researchers in the field of wellbeing in the later years, Stanford University psychologist Laura Carstensen, informs us in her 2007 article, *Growing Old or Living Long: Take Your Pick*, that, although we face a number of adversities that accompany aging, our sense of wellbeing seems to be largely unaffected. In fact, most older adults enjoy high levels of affective wellbeing and emotional stability well into their 70's and 80's. In fact, it appears that, as noted earlier, people are much happier by the time they reach 60 than they were in their 30's. It is suggested that individuals experience more life satisfaction as age increases because, with passing time and shrinking time horizons, they spend more hours and days in activities that contribute to their wellbeing instead of pursuing goals that are expected to pay off in the future. Further, it is likely that happiness increases slightly with age because, as time goes by, people become more realistic, realising that their expectations were probably set too high in those younger years. Put simply, because older people are more aware of mortality, they try to focus on things that contribute to their current happiness.

Research to understand the psychological and emotional processes of aging is essential to creating a society in which the elderly can thrive.

Laura Carstensen.

A sense of control has been repeatedly identified as an important factor in the wellbeing of older adults. Ute Kunzmann and other German researchers reported in their 2002 article, *Perceiving Control: A Double-edged Sword in Old Age*, that when elderly people perceive that they have control over decisions affecting their life, they have high emotional wellbeing. In contrast, for those who see that others have such control, there is a high risk that they will feel depressed and demeaned – unless of course there is a social confidence that they will benefit from others' control (e.g. "When I want them to, other people will help to arrange for good things to happen."). Further to these findings, Australian psychologists Robert Cummins and Helen Nistico, in their 2002 paper, *Maintaining Life Satisfaction: The Role of Positive Cognitive Bias*, focussed on the dilemma over control facing the elderly. They found that, although the degree of control that people have over their circumstances obviously decreases in advancing years, their happiness is increasingly dependent upon having this control as they move into old and very old age.

For those who are wondering how they can prepare psychologically for the challenge of their later years, the advice given by the Mexican spiritual teacher Don Juan to the well-known writer Carlos Castanada, is worth reflecting on:

> *Know that you have absolutely no power at all over the events that will impact on your life, but live as if you have absolute power.*

Allied to this is the Serenity Prayer, said to be composed by the American theologian Reinhold Niebuhr in the early 1940's and adopted by Alcoholics Anonymous:

God grant me the serenity to accept the things I cannot change,
Courage to change the things I can,
And wisdom to know the difference.

Research studies into how aging affects subjective wellbeing (that is, a sense of happiness, of interest in the world) have found that it is related to how well the older person can adapt to their circumstances. Neuronal plasticity, or the capability of the brain to adapt to new requirements, declines slowly during what is called the Third Age (65 to 80 years), then rapidly during the Fourth Age (starting at 80 or 85 years), the last years of adulthood. As such, with a decreasing ability to adapt, along with declining physical and cognitive robustness, the sense of wellbeing for many of the oldest of the old is unfortunately very poor or non-existent.

Whether older persons can cope with stressful situations, function well, and maintain their wellbeing appears to depend upon the resources they have. Several key ways of adapting used by older people have been identified:

◇ Coping

Coping involves managing stressful situations, dealing with finding some meaning in their plight, and managing the stress resulting from these situations. Older persons tend to use *emotion-focussed coping,* a strategy that refers to reminding oneself of the positive aspects of an adverse event (e.g. "I am ready for this, whatever it may be."), or controlling the symptoms of stress (e.g. relaxation exercises, mindful walking, confiding in others, etc.) rather than trying to manage the stressful situation itself.

Those who regard a threatening or stressful situation as challenging and who actively seek to find solutions are less likely to experience depression. However, some of the stressors experienced by older people, such as frailty and chronic health problems, are not easily modified by problem-solving; thus older persons may cope by bringing some meaning into the situation (e.g. "This is happening so that I can learn more patience."), or restructuring their priorities (e.g. "Finding inner happiness is now more important to me than trying to please others.").

Older persons also cope by comparing their situation with others, often using family and friends as reference points (e.g. "I'm not as badly off as Uncle Joe. He's lost both of his legs because of diabetes. At least I can still walk a few steps."). This strategy helps them to see that hardships are not aimed solely at themselves, but also imposed on others close to them.

◇ Social support

Social support includes both material and socio-emotional assistance provided by families, friends, neighbours, and volunteers or through private or governmental services, including religious organizations and centres for seniors.

Social support may also soften the adverse effects of various stressors common to aging. Researchers point out, however, that the effectiveness of social support depends on the situation, the person, and his or her needs; thus, goodness-of-fit is essential. Unneeded, unwanted, or the wrong type of support may reduce a person's independence or self esteem.

◇ Sense of control

Many older people are able to maintain a sense of mastery over the circumstances of their lives and this sense extends into late life as a resource important to wellbeing. Those working with older persons can reinforce this sense of control by respecting their right to make decisions or to initiate, withdraw, or terminate treatment.

Older Persons Functioning at a High Level

In their 1999 book, *Successful Aging,* gerontology researchers John Rowe and Robert Kahn describe their series of studies on older persons who are functioning at a high level. They identified three prominent characteristics common to those elderly who were aging 'successfully':

1. Low risk of disease and disease-related disability
2. High mental and physical function
3. Active engagement with life

The researchers found that those who maintained optimal physical and mental health through later life had a combination of all three of the above. More recently, university psychologist Martha Crowther and colleagues wrote in a 2002 issue of *The Gerontologist* that a range of research studies have identified an important addition to the above markers for successful aging: that of *positive spirituality* which they define using aspects of both religion and spirituality. They say that:

> *Positive spirituality involves a developing and internalized personal relation with the sacred or transcendent that is not bound by race, ethnicity, economics or class and promotes the wellness and welfare of self and others.*
>
> *Positive spiritual beliefs provide a cognitive framework that reduces stress and increases purpose and meaning in the face of illness. Spiritual activities like prayer and being prayed for may reduce the sense of isolation and increase the patient's sense of control over illness and disease.*

Theorists and researchers in gerontology agree that the ideal way to age into the later years is for an individual – throughout their adult life – to learn how to confront adverse situations not as a passive victim but as an actor drawing on resources developed over the course of their life. The development of such pro-active and positive coping skills over many years prepares them for the young-old and old-old periods of their life. Being readied in this way, stressors, such as those that involve health and the deaths of loved ones, can be reduced by finding a higher purpose and meaning underlying the loss, accepting and reaching out for social support, and retaining a sense of mastery over significant changes (e.g. "Regardless of what happens to me, I can choose how to think, feel and react.").

Mental Health in Old Age

Most people think of the elderly in terms of loss and decline. However, there is a growing body of research that many older people experience feelings of wellbeing, autonomy, togetherness and security, all of which they manage through self-care and inner strength.

However, despite this overall positive picture of mental health in the later years, the research studies show that the elderly, in common with other age groups, can experience a range of mental health concerns. These can affect thoughts, feelings, and behaviour; and influence family and social relations. The major mental health problems amongst older people include dementia, anxiety disorders, major depression and bipolar disorder, and abuse of alcohol or prescription drugs. Psychotic illnesses such as schizophrenia, delusional disorders, and paranoia are less common. Other mental health problems that may affect older adults include adjustment and sleep disorders.

Accepting the Aging Process

Reunion with our innate Peaceful Mind and Open Heart is possible if we can regard the closing years of our life as the ultimate initiation. In these Third and Fourth Ages, we encounter unexpected, unfamiliar, and unknowable moments that remind us that we are a sacred mystery that is being made manifest. If we can understand what is required of us at this stage, we are blessed with an unsurpassed opportunity to develop and embody peace, love, wisdom and beauty. There are limitless possibilities for us to restore, renew, and heal ourselves. And, because of our generation's increased longevity, for the first time in history we also have the opportunity to create a map for finding the Treasure of unshakeable inner peace, lasting happiness, and spiritual fulfilment that future generations can use as they enter their own later years.

How can we meet the challenges and opportunities of the closing years of our life? How can we do it better than has been done before? We can commit ourselves to developing increased integrity, depth and character within ourselves; to fostering gratitude; and to rediscovering our innate Human Values of Love, Truth, Peace, Right Conduct and Non-violence. If we choose to grow and embrace ever-deepening love, peace and wisdom, we must be willing to go through an ongoing self-transformation. In this way we can evolve into wise and engaged elders who provide meaningful contributions to other individuals, families, organizations, and communities. Regardless of what calamities, losses and impairments befall us, may our journey light a new path for future generations. May we be among those illustrious ones who will reclaim and model the dignity, grace and authentic power that true elderhood confers.

Once we accept our limits,
we go beyond them.

Albert Einstein

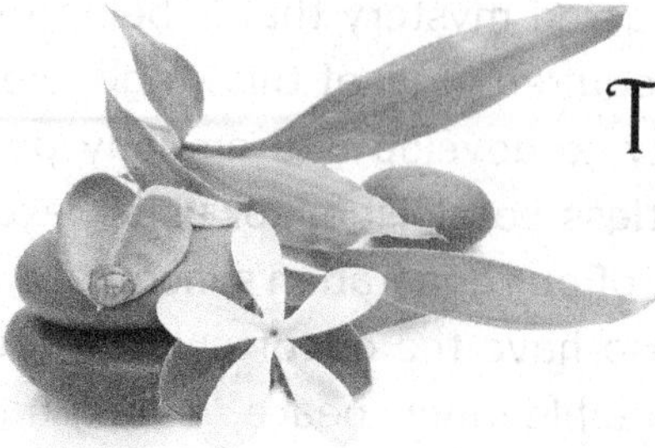

The Practice

EXERCISES FOR REJUVENATING THE POWER OF GRATITUDE

Exercise 1:
Why Be Grateful?

Many of us fear the onset of old age because it involves loss in so many forms: loss of control, loss of a loved one, loss of mental skills and physical fitness, and so on. Whether we are already in our elderly years or they still lie ahead of us, we are at an advantage if we can develop the habit of gratitude – a grateful heart is a joyful heart, whereas the attitude of 'I wish this wasn't happening to me' brings only depression, hardship and even ill-health. Understanding the value of being grateful is the first step towards maximising life satisfaction.

How can I do this exercise?

◇ Read the following sayings about gratitude and select the one that feels best for you:

1. When the heart begins to open in gratitude, it's like turning the water pot right side up to catch the life-giving rain.
2. Training the mind to be thankful – for gain or loss, praise or censure, success or failure – is a vital ingredient for inner peace.
3. To avoid thinking we are left out, disadvantaged, unfortunate,

we need to be ever-thankful for the multitude of riches our lives provide.

4. When we give thanks for everything, both good and bad, it is as if the sun comes out on a grey and cloudy day.
5. When we discover the uplifting power of gratitude, we find ourselves cherishing every moment of being alive.

◇ Having chosen your favourite saying, repeat it or write it out many times until you can recite it automatically at any time.

◇ For one week spend 3 to 5 minutes every night before going to sleep repeating your favourite reason for being grateful.

◇ Write to a friend, telling them what you are discovering about being more grateful.

Exercise 2:

How Can the Bad be Good?

How can we give thanks for what seems like a loss? For an answer to this we look at Nature all around: so perfect, balanced and pure. Every event in Nature, whether growth or decay, abundance or loss, contributes to this ideal scene.

When we feel lost, battered, defeated and wronged, there is always an example from Nature which can remind us to remember that our higher Self – the sun behind the clouds; the diamond hidden in the mud – is indestructible and ever-content.

How can I do this exercise?

- Find 3 or 4 examples in Nature where something good comes out of a calamity (e.g. the burning, cutting and crushing of the sugar-cane results in sugar so sweet).
- Look back over your life to recall a very difficult time or event which led eventually to it being a gift (e.g. you were ridiculed and this prompted you to increase your belief in yourself).
- Write this out in a special Gratitude Journal.
- Over the next few weeks and months, look for more examples in your life where good came out of adversity. Write each one in your Gratitude Journal.

<u>Exercise 3:</u>

Gratitude Journals

We know from the university research of Robert Emmons that people who keep gratitude journals feel better about their lives in many ways: they sleep better at night, are more positive, have better health, and they make progress towards important goals.

How can I do this exercise?

- Buy a good quality journal for your Gratitude Journal.
- Write down 20 things you feel grateful for right now. Begin each one with, "I am grateful for ... "
- Read through these every day, reflecting on each one, and adding one or two more that come to mind, until the list seems to cover every aspect of your life.
- Most people write in their Gratitude Journals just before going to sleep. The idea is to reflect on the day and write down five things or events you can give thanks for. It could be a letter from a friend, less

pain than yesterday, a kind word from someone, the sight of a butterfly or a rainbow, or some great music or a book, whatever comes to mind.

Exercise 4:

Breathing in, I Feel Grateful

Linking words of gratitude with the breath is a powerful way to develop the habit of thankfulness. Why? Because every breath is an extraordinary gift – without it we would lose this life.

How can I do this exercise?

- ◇ Bring your attention to your breath, and keep returning it there as well as you can.

- ◇ Say quietly in your mind, in time with each breath, "Breathing in, I give thanks for this breath," and, "Breathing out, I give thanks for this breath."

- ◇ Do this for 5 to 10 breaths.

- ◇ Now, still expressing gratitude for your breath, reduce the words in your mind to 'Thank you' each time you breathe in, and again each time you breathe out.

- ◇ Do this for 10 to 20 breaths.

- ◇ Now, each time you breathe in, say to yourself, "I give thanks for being alive," and, each time you breathe out, "I give thanks for being alive."

◇ Do this for 5 to 10 breaths.

◇ Now, still feeling gratitude for being alive, reduce the words in your mind to 'Thank you' each time you breathe in, and again each time you breathe out.

◇ Do this for 10 to 20 breaths.

◇ You might like to explore saying 'Thank you' with each in- and out-breath while you are walking, driving, riding in a bus or train, or waiting in a queue.

◇ If you want to develop the habit of gratitude so that it becomes automatic, in any situation, for the rest of your life, you can experiment with saying 'Thank you' in time with your breath for other gifts we can easily take for granted: for your body, whether healthy or in pain; for your mind, whether clear or fading; for moments of happiness, friendship and compassion; for the view out of the window; for the sight of a bird flying in the sky; for your loved ones and for those who provoke you; anything you like.

Those who knew Albert Einstein said that he repeated 'Thank you' hundreds of times every day.

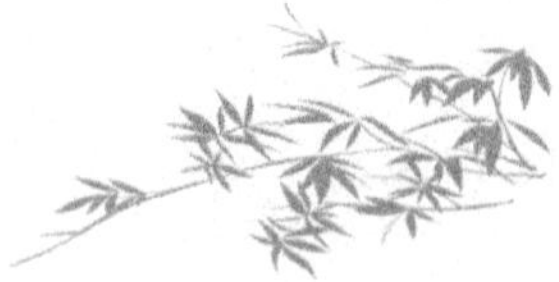

Exercise 5:

Letters of Gratitude

How can I do this exercise?

- ◇ Once every week, send a note of gratefulness to someone who enriched your life in some way. They could be a friend or relative, the author of a book, or a teacher or neighbour from years ago.

- ◇ If the person is deceased, you can write a gratitude note, keep it for a while, and then burn it in reverence.

- ◇ You might like to write a short note or poem of gratitude to an aspect of Nature that gives you joy, contentment or courage. For example, "Beloved clouds in the sky, you give me a new colourful painting every day ... Thank you. Thank you."

At times, our own light goes out and is rekindled by a spark from another person. Each of us has cause to think with deep gratitude of those who have lighted the flame within us.

Albert Schweitzer

Chapter 9

The Neuroscience of Aging

The knowledge that we acquire early in life
tends to be stored throughout life.
As we age, we develop a history of life experiences,
and we see the end of processes as well as the beginnings.

Jordan Grafman

Widespread concern about the rising incidence of brain disease over the past thirty years, coupled with the development of sophisticated brain imaging technologies, has spurred an avalanche of research into the neuroscience of the aging brain. We know that the way in which the different regions of the brain interact with each other and the coalition of neurotransmitter systems is common to us all, and yet there are enormous individual differences that account for the variability in how well we age.

We are all aging and some of us will find ourselves either caring for those with cognitive and physical impairments, or facing the challenge of being afflicted ourself, or both. The future can appear to be quite daunting in this regard. However, gaining some understanding of the psycho-socio-neuro-biological mechanisms influencing this human form that we reside in allows us to enter the field with both the dispassion of the explorer and the compassion of the carer. To that end, some central research findings are described below.

The Changes in the Brain

◇ Brain mass

It has been widely found that the volume of the brain and/or its weight declines with age at a rate of around 5 percent per decade after age 40. Beginning in about the sixth or seventh decade of life, brain mass shrinks steadily – particularly in such areas as the frontal lobe and the hippocampus.

Although the shrinking of the brain's grey matter is often reported to stem from the death of neuronal cells (specialized cells transmitting nerve impulses), losing perhaps 30,000 to 50,000 neurons a day from the brain and nervous system, a number of researchers say that a decline in the volume rather than the number of neurons could be the main reason for the shrinking of the brain with age.

As noted above, the brain mass atrophy that comes with aging is most pronounced in the frontal lobes and the medial temporal lobe where the hyppocampus is located. A decline in functioning of the hyppocampus can reduce a person's ability to move information from short-term to long-term memory (shown as difficulty in recalling details of events), and to remember where they have been and how to get where they are going (spatial navigation).

Loss of neuron volume in the frontal lobes may account for slower movements in the elderly, for the intrusion of socially-unacceptable speech and behaviour in some, and for others a reduced ability to see ahead to the consequences of their present actions. With the reduction in brain mass that accompanies all aging, particularly into the 70's and 80's, any or all of the above deficits are possible, although the severity of the difficulties varies widely over individuals.

Apart from the need to develop a compassionate understanding of the challenges facing the elderly, it is valuable to consider our own future – that is, to imagine the worst and to prepare psychologically for that possibility, and to take whatever steps we can in our pre-elderly years to nurture the health of the brain. Facing such fears in ourselves allows us to be more present and open-hearted with those who are struggling with the more severe forms of brain mass loss.

◇ Cortical density

The heavily-ridged outer surface of the brain undergoes modest thinning. This does not reflect widespread neuron loss but is probably due to the steadily declining density of synaptic connections, which begins around age 20. Fewer thread-like fibers to send and receive nerve signals in the cortex may contribute to slower cognitive processing.

◇ White matter

Many studies have linked aging with a decrease in white matter, the bundles of axons that carry nerve signals between brain cells. There are some indications that the deterioration of the white matter is caused by damage to the myelin sheath. This sheath consists of glial-cell extensions that wrap around the axon and enable it to conduct nerve impulses more quickly. With aging, the lengths of the axons seem to shorten, and myelin shrinks. Since myelin improves nerve transmission efficiency, its loss may slow processing. Scientists have correlated these changes with the reduced cognitive function that is observed in the course of aging.

For those wishing to engage in their own preventative measures to retard the rate of any deterioration in white matter – and the consequent decline in cognitive function – the research about myelin reported by Daniel Coyle in his 2009 book, *The Talent Code*, is worth considering.

As noted in some detail earlier in Chapter 5, the thickness of the microscopic myelin sheath that forms around neurons' axons – so as to increase conduction speed from one neuron to another neuron across the synapse – grows when a neuronal circuit is repeatedly activated. Daniel Coyle presents persuasive evidence that perseverance and struggle to master new skills and overcome obstacles is the ideal generator for growing myelin.

◇ Neurotransmitter systems

The main function of the many billions of neurons in our brain is to communicate with each other across tiny junctions called synapses. When a neuron fires, an electrochemical wave ripples down its axon, the microscopic fibre extending towards other neurons. When this happens, tendrils at the end of the neuron's axon expel a burst of molecules into the synapses – the connections – it makes with other neurons. Each tendril contains about 200 little bubbles (vesicles) that are full of neurotransmitters (mostly serotonin and dopamine). Every time the neuron fires, five to ten vesicles spill open and neurotransmitters are sent across to other receiving neurons, either inhibiting or exciting them to fire. Research has identified over 100 different neurotransmitters that are floating around the brain, waiting to be gathered into the vesicles ready to be used for neural transmission.

The aging brain generates less of these chemical messengers and has fewer receptors to lock onto them. Decreased dopamine, acetylcholine, serotonin, and norepinephrine activity may contribute to declining memory and cognition and to increased depression among older people.

The neurotransmitters most often researched with regard to aging are dopamine and serotonin. Dopamine is involved with rewards and attention, and promotes approach behaviour. What happens is that dopamine-releasing neurons become more active when we encounter things that are linked to rewards in the past, because they could offer rewards in the future. If the rewards are not forthcoming, dopamine levels drop which is experienced by us as a dissatisfaction or discontent. When the aging brain produces less dopamine, depression can descend upon the person.

Whether the levels of dopamine drop mostly because the elderly person is experiencing the loss of so many sought-after experiences, or because of age-degeneration, is not yet clear.

Regardless of the cause, it is incumbent upon us to find ways of increasing dopamine levels in the elderly, perhaps by using reminders from the past that once brought great joy. The SWAMI Home in Singapore regularly takes residents into a Reminiscence Room where they can touch now-antique objects from the period of their childhood. In a number of nursing homes for the incapacitated aged in the USA and Canada, audio recordings of each person's favourite music from their pre-illness years are played into residents' headphones, producing quite remarkable results. It was in 2014 that Dan Cohen founded the non-profit *Music & Memory* organisation that brings playlists of preferred music (associated with personal memories) into the lives of those struggling with Alzeihmer's and other forms of dementia, using MP3 players and related digital audio systems. Featured in the movie, *Alive Inside*, this form of music therapy can help to decrease difficult behaviours, improve communication, reconnect with loved ones, and increase overall quality of life.

For ourselves, as preparation for a possible future when dopamine levels are reduced, we can increase our search for that lasting happiness that is not dependent upon outside sources, but is ever-present within, until we can imagine being alone, with all familiar forms of entertainment removed, and feel content and happy, like sitting next to a warm fire on a cold winter's night.

◇ Pre-frontal cortex

As noted in earlier chapters, the pre-frontal cortex sets goals, makes plans, directs actions, and shapes emotions, in part by guiding and sometimes inhibiting the limbic system, which is central to emotion and motivation. The pre-frontal cortex plays a vital role in relation to the growth and expression of virtues – all of which are subsumed under the umbrellas of the five universal Human Values of Love, Truth, Peace, Right Conduct and Non-violence .

The pre-frontal cortex shows notable changes with aging. At a structural level, there is evidence of atrophy, both in the grey matter and in the white matter. As noted earlier, the grey matter declines may reflect reductions in the number of cells (due to cell death) or may be a sign of neuronal shrinkage. The white matter changes reflect axonal abnormalities, and may result in slowed neurotransmission. It is likely that these white matter changes may be the cause of the cognitive slowing that accompanies healthy aging.

Research studies have shown that much can be done to offset deterioration in the pre-frontal cortex. Using detected image segmentation of high-resolution brain scans, it has been shown that regular physical exercise, the practice of mindfulness, and development of empathy can help to grow more neurons and white matter in the pre-frontal cortex.

Daniel Siegel, in his 2009 book, *The Mindful Brain: Reflection and Attunement in the Cultivation of Well-Being,* explains the neuroscience governing how mindful awareness practices can change the function and structure of the brain, mostly in the pre-frontal cortex.

He notes that Buddhist monks who have practised mindful awareness (one-pointed attention on, say, the breath) for thousands of hours have a notably 'thicker' pre-frontal cortex.

The self-discipline that is required in mindfulness practice to shift attention repeatedly away from the more-entrenched, habitual patterns of neural firing (to do with a restless body and a wandering mind) cultivates the growth of new specialised brain cells that form linkages to thousands of other neurons. The abandoned cells gradually die and the new ones receiving attention multiply, giving us the rewards of : improved attention and concentration, enhanced work and sport performance, improved control over strong negative emotions, reduction in stress levels, a boost in the body's immune system, and so much more. We will return to the benefits of mindfulness for aging in Chapter 11.

◇ Amygdala

The amygdala helps detect potentially emotionally-relevant stimuli – relevant because they are novel, pose a threat, or are goal-relevant – and then modulates other brain systems to enhance attention and memory for those stimuli. It is clearly involved in anxiety and fear, but also plays a part in positive affect and motivation.

Studies indicate that, in older adults, the amygdala shows relatively little decline in structure or function in normal aging. Rather, it is the reduced functioning of those other parts of the brain (e.g. pre-frontal cortex) responsible for vetting and inhibiting impulses from the amygdala that can make life difficult for some elderly people. The ability to censor and regulate such impulses plays an essential role in our ability to fit in with social norms and ensure moral behaviour. When a person loses the ability to fully regulate input from the amygdala, this can lead to social isolation and loneliness because of their unwitting offensive behaviour.

Compassion for the plight of those elderly so afflicted is required. Loving understanding can ease their pain significantly. Also, we can more readily be non-judgmental of their behaviour if we recognise the possibility that, unless we have fully expunged all of our lower (reptilian) impulses by then, we ourselves could be challenged with such uncontrollable impulses if we were to be beset with such a severe deterioration in the brain.

◇ Insular cortex

The insular cortex (or insula) is an embedded part of the cerebral cortex that plays a significant role in bodily self-awareness. The insula is also involved in a range of functions to do with emotion and the autonomic nervous system (for homeostasis), including: perception, motor control, self-awareness, cognitive functioning, empathy, hand-eye motor control, swallowing, speech, risk and uncertainty processing, and interpersonal experience.

Findings regarding aging adults indicate that the insula shows moderate age-related decline with notable individual differences. Insula deterioration can result in apathy, lack of empathy, confused decision-making and inaccurate time perception. The apathy is probably due to the inability of the brain to interpret bodily states (e.g. changes in breathing, specific muscular tensions) that are triggered by emotional events. That is, the person is not aware of any emotional feeling even though his body might be reacting in the habitual emotional way.

To address decline, there are promising indications from neuroscience that regular meditation increases grey matter (number of neurons) in the insular cortex as well as other areas of the brain. Also, it is established that exercise increases both grey and white matter throughout the brain.

We have explored briefly just a few of the mechanisms that play a major role in the aging brain for determining the quality of our thinking, memory, emotions and behaviour. Each one of these is the subject of ongoing, extensive research, both individually and collectively. In due course, researchers will turn their attention towards those interrelationships between heart, mind and brain that are relevant to what does not change: that vantage point from which the higher Self calmly observes even the most dramatic changes without departing from its essential attribute of pure, lasting, authentic happiness - Peaceful Mind, Open Heart.

Old age is not a defeat, but a victory, not a punishment but a privilege. It can be regarded not as the age of stagnation or decline, but as the age of opportunities for inner growth.

A test of a people is how it behaves toward the old. It is easy to love children. Even tyrants and dictators make a point of being fond of children. But the affection and care for the old, the incurable, the helpless are the true gold mines of a culture.

Abraham Joshua Heschel

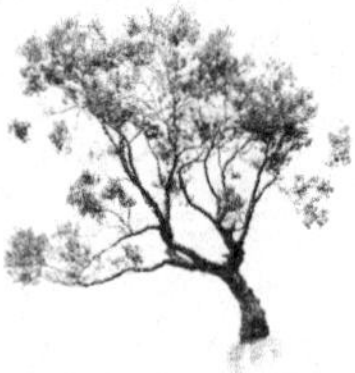

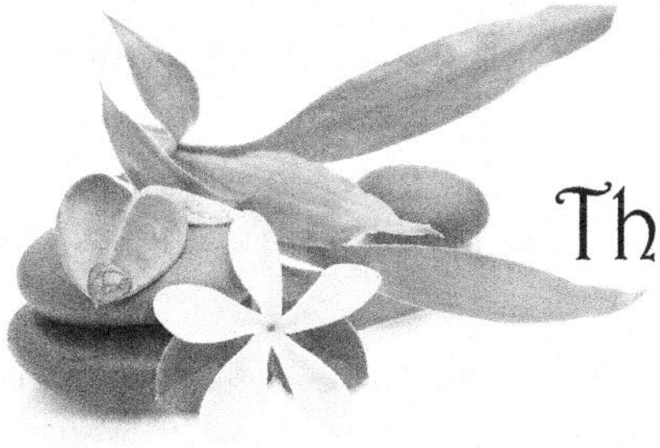

The Practice

EXERCISES FOR GROWING THE BRAIN

The brain's ability to manage the vast complexities of human thinking, feeling, behaving, remembering and discriminating is dependent upon an even more vast array of neurobiological components in the brain that function at barely measurable speeds in microscopic dimensions. The exercises to follow are derived from research findings concerning self-initiated interventions that can 'grow' the three most significant brain elements that decline with aging: grey matter (neurons), white matter (myelin) and neurotransmitters.

Because neuroscience is not yet able to delineate precisely which exercises are best for each element, what is offered here are those that are believed to be positive in their effect, in a general sense.

<u>Exercise 1:</u>
Physical Exercise

How can I do this exercise?

- ◇ As a first step, limit sedentary relaxation periods (e.g. watching TV) to a minimum.
- ◇ Secondly, endeavour to do all household and gardening chores (cooking, cleaning, mowing, weeding, etc.) yourself, instead of engaging others to do them for you.

◇ Make up an exercise program that involves you in brisk walking, swimming or bicycle riding as much as your body allows, building up your strength gradually.

◇ Join a class for aerobic exercising, something that requires you to breathe deeper and increases heart rate, ideally under the guidance of a professional.

◇ To improve hand-eye coordination and reaction time reflexes, consider getting involved in sports such as badminton or table tennis.

◇ The great 19th century yogi of India, Swami Vivekananda, recommended that we spend 5 to 10 minutes in the morning, breathing according to the counting ratio of: Inhalation (2 sec.), Hold Breath (8 sec.), Exhalation (4 sec.). With practice you might build up gradually to: In (4 sec.), Hold (16 sec.), Out (8 sec.). This oxygenates the brain without hyperventilating.

Exercise 2:

Mental Exercises

How can I do this exercise?

◇ Many forms of mental exercise have been recommended by neuroscientists, including: crossword puzzles; learning a language; remembering affirmations, prayers or uplifting poems; avoiding using a calculator when adding up numbers; reading out loud.

◇ Of particular value are those exercises requiring intense concentration, for example:

1. Recite as quickly as possible the regular ascending series of numbers:
   2, 4, 6, 8, up to 100; and then, 3, 6, 9, 12, up to 99; and so on, beginning with 4, then 5, then 6, etc.

2. The same in descending order, first by 2's, then 3's, and so on until by 9's:
   That is, by 2's: 100, 98, 96 ... and so on.
   Then, by 3's: 100, 97, 94 ... and so on.
   And so on until by 9's: 100, 91, 82 ... and so on.
3. Recite two ascending series together, using 2's and 3's.
   That is: 2, 3; 4, 6: 6, 9; ... to 66, 99.
4. Recite two descending series together from 100, using 2's and 3's.
   That is: 98, 97; 96, 94; 94, 91; ... and so on.
5. Recite three ascending series together, using 2's, 3's and 5's.
   That is: 2, 3, 5; 4, 6, 10; 6, 9, 15; ... and so on.
6. Recite three descending series together, from 100 using 2's, 3's and 5's .
   That is: 98, 97, 95; 96, 94, 90; 94, 91, 85; ... and so on.

◇ Recite the alphabet backwards.

◇ Memorise accurately some four-lined verse (e.g. Jack and Jill ...)

◇ Progress through the verse, spelling each word backwards.

◇ Begin to learn a new language, spending at least 30 minutes every day on the task.

◇ Obtain a Thesaurus. Select a word at random and rote learn every synonym given for that word. On the next day, recite the synonyms for the word as best you can, and relearn until you can recite them all. Then select a new word and rote learn its synonyms, and so on.

◇ Select a poem that has a special wisdom relevant for you and rote learn it. Reflect on it each day as you recite it, gaining deeper understanding and insights. After perhaps one week, select another poem, and so on.

Exercise 3:
Mindfulness Exercises

There will be a number of mindfulness exercises in The Practice at the end of Chapter 11. However, you might like to try this simple one to do with counting the breaths.

How can I do this exercise?

- Find a quiet place. Sit or lie straight. Bring the attention to the breath.
- Each time you breathe in, add another (number) one. That is, counting the breaths.
- If your mind wanders away from the task and you forget to count, return to counting the breaths, beginning at number one again.
- At first try, you might get up to 5 or 6, or even more. Each time you forget and start again, you'll be competing against yourself, steadily improving your concentration, until you can reach 30, 40 or 50 breaths before you forget to count.

Creating a joint venture between head and heart
puts a power pack behind your goals.
Getting your head in sync with your heart
and harnessing the power of coherence
gives you the energy efficiency you need
to achieve changes that haven't been possible before.
The head can notice what things need to change,
but the heart provides the power and direction
to actually bring about the changes.

Doc Childre and Howard Martin

Chapter 10

The Unchanging Self in the Ever-changing Flow of Life

Through our eyes, the universe is perceiving itself.
Through our ears, the universe is listening to its harmonies.
We are the witnesses through which
the universe becomes conscious of its glory,
of its magnificence.

Alan Watts

Because of the rapid elongation of human life span over this past century there are now a disproportionate number of elderly people in the technologically advanced countries such as the USA, the EU, China, Japan and elsewhere. Perhaps prompted by this dramatic growth of an aging population there has been an explosion of research during the past 20 years into what happens to us as we age.

Naturally, we would like to know what changes will take place as we enter into our greying and then closing years. Will we become sad, bitter and lonely? Will our minds and bodies become a liability? Or will we have the opportunity, now that we are relatively free of our householder responsibilities, to reflect, explore, and grow in wisdom, equanimity, happiness, tolerance and compassion?

As noted in a previous chapter, apart from some obvious slowing down of some physical and mental functions, the psychoneurological research shows that, in general, older adults maintain the ability to be positive about life and to minimise or let go of intrusive negative emotions. In her paper, *The Affective Neuroscience of Aging,* psychologist Mara Mather cites over 200 published studies in her extensive review of the research exploring what happens to the brain and the emotions of people as they age.

The general conclusion to be drawn from all of the relevant research, both psychological and neurophysiological, is that two of the main organs in the brain that are responsible for emotional reactivity, control and balancing of mood – the pre-frontal cortex (parts of it) and the amygdala – are not reduced in size or in their ability to function well. Mather says,

> *The relative lack of decline in core emotion-related brain regions likely plays a key role in explaining older adults' well-maintained emotional functioning, in particular the ability to maintain positive affect and minimize negative affect in everyday life.*

Some researchers into the effects of aging have proposed that the reason for the relative constancy of emotional balance over the years is a genetic predisposition to be happy or unhappy. That is, a person's *subjective well-being* or SWB (their subjective self-assessment of the quality of their lives, including both the range and balance of their emotions, and also their mental or cognitive activity and judgements) is fairly well set over their lifetime, with fluctuations but always returning to the same baseline or stable *Set Point* for their SWB measure.

In his 2000 book, titled *Happiness: The Nature and Nurture of Joy and Contentment,* David Lykken reviews much of the research in this field, including his own longitudinal studies with twin pairs, and goes on to advocate the importance of avidly seeking experiences that can push us beyond our happiness Set Points (e.g. doing the cooking vs watching the cooking channel on TV). If, as David Coyle recommends in his book about habits and the growth of myelin in the brain (see earlier), we can 'set the bar higher' than we have been used to doing, it is likely that we will not only improve the efficiency of our brain functioning but also lift our SWB steadily beyond our Set Point, our genetic predisposition.

Since it is common for people's SWB to keep returning to its Set Point, it could be that most of us seldom move too far out of our comfort zone. Perhaps the reason for this population-wide stasis is that very few are aware of their true potential, their higher Self or Soul, clothed in the lustre of the lofty and noble Human Values.

Throughout all of the research exploring what changes and what remains as we age, there is scant recognition of the unchanging Self which, regardless of the elevation or decay of the human form and its functions, is ever-content, ever-pure, ever-blissful and soaked in Love. Rather, there are neurological explanations as to why elderly people are more or less happy than younger ones, as if forgetting that, not only does the brain change the mind, the mind also moulds, sculpts and grows the brain.

From our point of view, the great value of aging is that our catalogue of errors and disappointments keeps filling up, leading to a heightened wisdom as to the value of mistakes, and a growing humility. Perhaps it is for this reason that old age can bring a growing contentment.

It is the contention of this thesis - the philosophy of the universal Human Values - that much can be added to the findings from modern neuroscience by attending to that Essence within us that never ages, never suffers and never dies.

What can we say of our Soul, our higher Self? Those who have gone before, who already know the Way, have left words to guide us. The great essayist of Abraham Lincoln's time, Ralph Waldo Emerson, described its mystery, power and glory in this way:

What we commonly call man, the eating, drinking, planting, counting man, does not, as we know him, represent himself, but misrepresents himself. Him we do not respect, but the soul, whose organ he is, would he let it appear through his action, would make our knees bend. When it breathes through his intellect, it is genius; when it breathes through his will, it is virtue; when it flows through his affection, it is love ... All reform aims, in some one particular, to let the soul have its way through us; in other words, to engage us to obey.

More recently, sometime before the year 2000, there was a BBC documentary about a nine-year-old boy in England who was dying of an incurable disease. Millions of people all over the world were deeply moved, uplifted, and changed somewhat by what they heard from the boy himself. He was responding to a question put to him by the interviewer who asked, "You don't seem to be concerned that you are dying. How is it that you can be so calm and cheerful even though you have been told by the doctors that you only have weeks to live?" The boy smiled and looked at the man as if he was puzzled by the question, as if he was thinking, "Don't you know? How come you don't know?" Then he smiled again and said, "Why should I be worried or frightened? Nothing will be happening to me. I'll just be leaving this body and getting into a different sort of body."

The television reporter still did not understand: "But you won't be alive anymore." to which the boy gave a longer answer. Patiently and respectfully, the boy said, "Look at it this way. When I go to bed tonight, I'll be getting out of these clothes and getting into my sleeping clothes. I'll still be me. I'll just be in different clothes." He paused for a few seconds, and then said, "This body that I'm in right now is like my day clothes. Sometime soon I'll be getting into a different body, which will be like my night clothes. Do you see what I mean?" The millions of people watching the show were profoundly moved. They believed him but were not sure why.

Most of the time we live and behave as if we are this human form with mind, feelings and personality. And so we usually fear the gradual or sudden decline of the body and its functions, the possibility of severe memory loss with aging, not being able to retain control over how we live if we are severely incapacitated, and so on. And, deep down, most of us fear death, finding it hard to imagine our body being buried in the ground or burnt in a furnace. We might ask, "Is this how it is meant to be; living as if decline, loss and death are to be feared?"

Without realising it, we have spent most our lives identifying with our experiences and circumstances and then coming to assume they are part of who we are. We have identified ourselves with a name, race, gender and nationality. We have identified ourselves with our knowledge, skills and occupations, and with what we think are our personality traits (funny, trustworthy, judgmental, etc.), and most of all we have assumed that we are our bodies, each one with its own shape, looks, weight, colour and fitness.

Many reasons have been offered over the centuries as to why we unwittingly hold on to thinking that we are these identities, one of them being that they give us a sense of security, believing they are the 'real me'. So often we've heard people say, when defending their right to be angry, stubborn, selfish or unforgiving, "But this is who I am. I've always been this way," little realising that these qualities are not who we are, anymore than the car that we drive around in is who we are.

Why is it that we feel so identified with these bodies that think, feel and move? Perhaps it is because we appear to gain happiness and also experience suffering (the absence of happiness) through this form, this body/mind complex.

As noted in earlier pages, the Human Values philosophy – which is identical to the perennial philosophy of Aldous Huxley, Ralph Waldo Emerson, the Sufis, Wayne Dyer and all those known as transcendentalists – asserts that pure, unbounded happiness already lies within us, and that the craving for sense indulgence, social recognition and all else that fades with time, is a clear indication that we've not yet realised who we really are, that we are our true Self, that which never fades, never grows old or infirm, and never dies. The Sanskrit poet Bhartrihari captures the pathos of this life-long yearning for union with things that do not last in his *Century of Verses on Renunciation:*

My face is graven with wrinkles
My head is marked with grey,
My limbs are withered and feeble -
My craving alone keeps its youth.

Saints and sages and the adored founders of the seven major religions all gave advice (to the effect) that, if we want to lessen our suffering and increase happiness, it is imperative that we assign more importance to seeking the ever-present Heaven within, rather than crave for ten thousand heavenly imitations that soon fade with time. Using different terminologies, they go on to say that the gates to this inner Treasure invite us to enter when we remember that our true Self is unchanging, immortal, ever-blissful, supremely loving, and beauty beyond compare – riches that are infinitely more valuable than anything we can experience in our worldly pursuit of happiness. As Swami Vivekananda said in one of his talks over one hundred years ago:

... all the pleasure we know is but a reflection, an atom, of that bliss that we get from touching our real nature.

Particularly amongst those who have suffered for so long, and equally so for those who insist that the pleasures offered by the world are real and sufficient, the most frequently-asked question on this topic would be: "But why should I believe that inexhaustible joy beyond measure lies waiting within me if I can't seem to feel any of it?" And an equally insistent objection is:

"Has science yet proved this? Can we measure this bliss that's supposed to be waiting inside us?" These concerns can be addressed with the *pearl diver* analogy. It goes like this:

> If we wanted to find out where to dive in the ocean for pearls, we'd go to the most successful pearl divers and ask them where to dive. Being sensible, we would dive exactly where they said to, and not go paddling around in the shallows instead. And who are the pearl divers? They are the great ones like Paramahamsa Ramakrishna, Lord Jesus, Ramana Maharshi, Meister Eckhart, The Dalai Lama and so forth. They all said, in effect, "If you want to find the real Treasure, the Kingdom of Heaven, it is here, only here, in the depths of yourself. Dive deep and you will find it."

The idea of a higher Self might be relatively easy to grasp at an intellectual level, but it's not always clear where to begin the search for this inner Treasure. Perhaps the most fruitful path is to begin with the unchanging nature of the true Self. The Self observes all changes, but never changes. The philosopher Dan Zahavi describes this ever-present Self in this way:

> *... the Self is some kind of ontologically independent invariant principle of identity that stands apart from, and above, the stream of changing experiences; something that remains unchanging from birth to death; something that remains entirely unaffected by language acquisition, social relationships, major life events, personal commitments, projects, and values, something that cannot develop or flourish nor be disturbed or shattered.*

It is difficult, perhaps impossible, to begin our search for the higher Self – our Peaceful Mind, Open Heart – if our mental faculties have become severely impaired through a brain disease or advanced aging. Recognising this possibility can prompt us to intensify our quest, while we are still able, for our unchanging Self.

Each time we take a step in this direction by becoming the Observer – the Witness – of all that is changing (our thoughts, sensations, environment, and so on), we will be rewiring our brain in ways that are more likely to give us a boat to sit in as we cross any turbulent seas on our journey into our closing years.

For those of a giving nature, perhaps of even more significance is that, if we can identify more with the ever-present Witness that we are, to that same extent we will be able to see through the clouds of anxiety, depression, anger, loneliness and confusion that might be covering the Sun in someone we are caring for. This is a great gift to anyone, regardless of the severity of their condition.

We can put ourselves in the shoes of the one who is lost and suffering. If a loving Soul looked through our veil of confusion and recognised their same Treasure lying untouched within us, we would feel so blessed, so loved, regardless of our condition.

If you feel lost, disappointed, hesitant, or weak, return to yourself, to who you are, here and now and when you get there, you will discover yourself, like a lotus flower in full bloom, even in a muddy pond, beautiful and strong.

Masaru Emoto

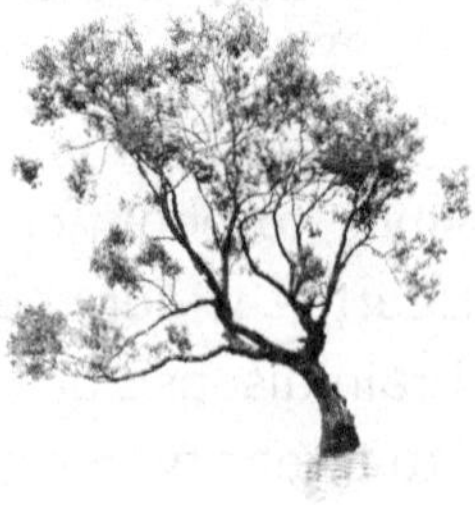

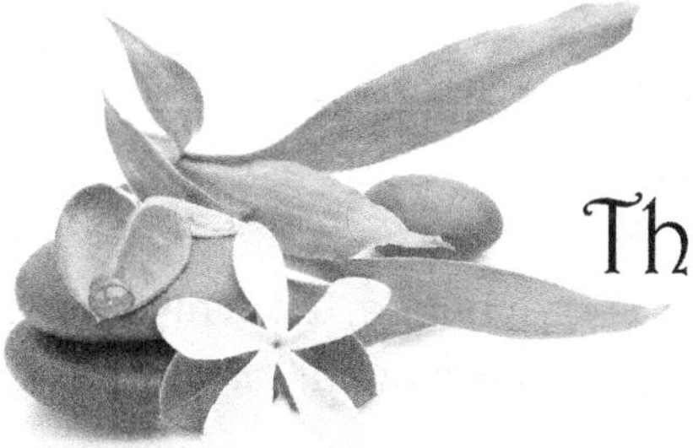

The Practice

EXERCISES TO REVEAL THE UNCHANGING SELF

These exercises are designed to help us begin a journey to connect with – identify with - our unchanging Self. This higher Self is Peaceful Mind, Open Heart; it is the five universal Human Values of Love, Truth, Peace, Right Conduct and Non-violence. As we come to experience for ourselves that we are the unchanging Self, this will help us to be steady, loving and joyful on our journey through life. And it will help us in our caring for others – knowing that who they really are (the true Self) is not in pain, but is observing the pain; is not confused and anxious, but is observing the confusion and anxiety. Such a wise, loving and detached attitude will be of immense value for each person we care for.

Exercise 1:
Retraining the Mind: Affirmations

Our pathway of awakening to the true Self is made easier if we can retrain the mind to think automatically in ways that support our journey.

How can I do this exercise?

◇ Read the following affirmations and select the one that feels right for you at this time:

1. The ocean knows that it is more than the dancing waves. The sky knows it is more vast than the few clouds that are constantly changing. And I am more than this changing body, thoughts, feelings, sensations and movements.
2. My body changes, and so too does everything I can see, hear, smell, taste and touch. My emotions change, and my thoughts change. But 'I' do not change. 'I' am observing all of these changes.
3. Who 'I' am, is changeless. 'I' am like the screen in a movie theatre upon which the movie of life is being projected. The fire in the movie does not burn the screen, nor does the flood make the screen wet. In the same way, 'I' am not affected by what this body thinks, feels and does. 'I' am the changeless 'I', ever- content, observing all of these changes.

◇ Write out your chosen affirmation in a special journal or print it on a card, and read it aloud every day, for as many days as feels right.

◇ Then if you wish, do this for another affirmation.

Exercise 2:
Retraining the Mind: Self as the Observer

How can I do this exercise?

◇ Make yourself comfortable in a quiet place.
◇ As you read each step, follow the instruction for 10 to 20 seconds.
◇ Notice your feet touching the floor.
◇ Notice what you can smell.
◇ Notice what you can taste.
◇ Notice what you can hear.

- ◇ Notice how you are breathing.
- ◇ Notice what your mind is telling you.
- ◇ Notice what you're feeling right now.
- ◇ Notice what your hands are touching.
- ◇ So there's a part of you that can notice everything you hear, touch, taste, smell and feel in any moment.
- ◇ Notice the thoughts you are having right now.
- ◇ Bring your awareness to your thoughts.
- ◇ Where do they seem to be located: above you, behind you, in front of you, inside you?
- ◇ Are your thoughts moving or still? If moving, in what direction? How fast?
- ◇ What form do your thoughts take? Are they more like pictures, or sounds, or words, or a mixture?
- ◇ As you observe your thoughts, be aware that you're observing them.
- ◇ There are your thoughts, and there is you observing them.
- ◇ If you observe your thoughts, you cannot be your thoughts.
- ◇ Whatever you can observe, whatever you are noticing, you cannot be that.
- ◇ You can ask, "Well then, who am 'I'?" and the only answer can be, "'I' am the Witness. 'I' am the ever-present Observer. 'I' am that which never changes."

<u>Exercise 3:</u>
Retraining the Mind: Who am I?

How can I do this exercise?

- ◇ Imagine that you are the big screen in a movie theatre. No movie is showing. There is only you, the screen.
- ◇ Think now of any scene from your past. It could be during your childhood, or any other time.

◇ Imagine that the scene you have recalled has been made into a movie, with you playing the role of yourself.
◇ Imagine again that you are the screen, but now the movie is being projected onto your surface. You'll need to be doing this part with your eyes closed. Remind yourself, "I am the screen, not the movie." Do this for 2 to 3 minutes, perhaps replaying the same movie a few times.
◇ Now choose a scene from the future, whatever you can imagine yourself being involved in.
◇ Imagine that the scene from the future has been made into a movie, with you playing the role of yourself.
◇ Imagine again that you are the screen, but not the movie being projected onto your surface. You'll need to be doing this part with your eyes closed. Remind yourself, "I am the screen, not the movie." Do this for 2 to 3 minutes, perhaps replaying the same movie a few times.
◇ Imagine again that you are the screen, but this time the movie being projected onto your surface is whatever is happening with you right now (that is, sitting or lying somewhere, wherever you are right now, following these instructions). You'll need to be doing this with your eyes closed. Do this for 2 to 3 minutes.
◇ As you go about your day after this, you can experiment with doing this for a few moments. That is, you are this screen that is within you and also everywhere. You are the ever-present Witness, and the movie of life is being projected onto you: what you can see and hear; your bodily sensations; whatever you are doing; your thoughts and feelings; everything that you are aware of; for all of these, you can say, "I am the screen, not the movie."
◇ With practice, this exercise can be particularly helpful in dealing with disturbing emotions. That is, keep repeating, "I am the screen, not the movie. I am the observer of this emotion. I am not the emotion."

Think of the rays of the sun shining into houses.
They are rays of the sun, and they are light,
but they are attached to the sun and not the houses.
When the sun sets, their light no more remains.
What we have to do, then, is to become the Sun itself,
so all fear of separation can forever be ended.

Jalaluddin Rumi

Part Four

Mindfully Embracing The Path of Aging

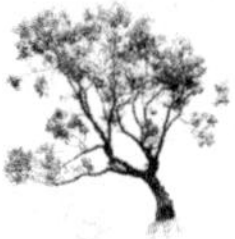

In the end, only three things matter:
How much you loved,
How gently you lived, and
How gracefully you let go
Of things not meant for you.

The Buddha

Chapter 11

The State of Mindfulness

Mindfulness means moment-to-moment, non-judgmental awareness. It is cultivated by refining our capacity to pay attention, intentionally, in the present moment, and then sustaining that attention over time as best we can.
In the process, we become more in touch with our life as it is unfolding.

Toni Bernhard

Even twenty-five years ago, the word 'mindfulness' was seldom heard, except perhaps when in the company of those psychologists and meditation teachers who were familiar with the words attributed to a Zen monk:

When I chop wood, I chop wood.
When I carry water, I carry water.

Now there are over six million internet responses to the search question of 'What is mindfulness?' Mindfulness is an idea whose time has arrived, after a wait of perhaps two thousand years or more. Certainly the notion of attending to what is happening in the present moment had been offered to the modern world well before the writings of Jon Kabat-Zinn and Thich Nhat Hanh, in particular, catapulted it into prominence during the 1990's, but only a few had responded.

Of the few, some were students of the ex-Harvard psychology professor, Richard Alpert, known later as Baba Ram Dass who wrote the 1967 inner-guide book for the New Age generation, *Be Here Now*; and others were ardent admirers of the writer A. R. Orage, a follower of the 1930's Russian-Armenian mystic G. I. Gurdjieff who advised all to 'remember to remember that you are asleep'. Orage gave a clear example of what we now call mindfulness in his *Psychological Exercises and Essays*:

> *Begin by trying to be aware of your movements and physical sensations while they are actually occurring ... Later try to notice your changing currents of feelings without, however, ceasing to be aware of your physical manifestations. Finally, try to become conscious of your streams of thinking; and include those observations with the previous observations or awareness of your physical and emotional life.*
>
> *The method is not introspective nor is it analysis. You are not required to think about it but only to be aware; and to be fully aware is to be fully conscious.*

These words of Orage and those earlier by Jon Kabat-Zinn describe an approach to living that allows us to become more aware of the fullness and richness of our moment-to-moment experiences in everyday life. When we awaken to the inner world of our body, mind and feelings, we become immersed in the mysterious beauty and perfection that permeates not only our lives and our surroundings, but those of all others as well, even when pain and suffering are demanding attention. The research findings are now there to support the idea that, if we can learn to pay attention, in the present moment, without drifting off into thoughts of past and future, or better or worse, our life satisfaction and feelings of authentic happiness will improve proportionally. We will find that our thoughts and feelings evolve to a higher level of love and wisdom, as will our interpersonal relationships with others.

Before we explore further the various ways of describing mindfulness and how to focus the mind in the moment, we might want to ask again the basic question: 'What is the mind?'

Almost all modern research on the mind has been concerned with its nature and function, rather than the more relevant issue for this Handbook's purpose: how to develop and enhance authentic happiness as we age? That is, how can we learn to become master of the mind instead of its slave? How can we retrain our mind so that it becomes an instrument for liberation rather than bondage, serenity instead of agitation, compassion rather than callous indifference, and so on?

Supported by a range of scientists from various disciplines, psychiatrist Daniel Siegel has often defined the mind as a process that regulates the flow of energy and information. He said that our human mind is both embodied and relational. 'Embodied' means that the mind involves a flow of information that occurs within the body, including the brain and nervous system.

The mind is 'relational' because our five senses are almost constantly responding to the appearance and behaviour of others as well as to our physical environment, and these inputs trigger the firing of neurons in the brain, which in turn adds information to what's in our mind.

Almost all of these modifications to the mind happen without our conscious awareness and so, lacking any discriminating oversight, the stream of incoming information merely goes towards reinforcing our established fears, prejudices and preferences.

In this way we interact with people, events and impressions as if we are highly-advanced, pre-programmed, biological robots, a condition which offers little opportunity for learning how to experience genuine life satisfaction and real, lasting happiness.

Mindfulness in its most general sense is about waking up from a life-on-automatic. With mindful awareness, the flow of energy and information that is our mind enters our conscious attention and we can both appreciate its content and also come to regulate its flow.

Mindful awareness, as we will see, actually involves more than just simply being aware. It involves being aware of aspects of the mind itself. Instead of being on automatic and not attending to the plethora of thoughts coming and going all day long (that is, being mindless, lacking mindful awareness), mindfulness helps us to be aware of (awaken to) the thoughts arriving, departing and returning with every moment, and, with this reflection on the mind, we make choice and change possible.

As you can see, the term *mindful awareness* is used interchangeably with *mindfulness*. How we focus attention plays a direct role in shaping the mind. When we develop a certain form of attention to our here-and-now experiences and to the nature of our mind itself, we create a special kind of awareness called mindfulness or mindful awareness.

Mindfulness, or direct experiencing in the present moment, has been described as a fundamental part of Buddhist, Christian, Hindu, Islamic, Jewish, and Taoist teaching for centuries.

In these religious traditions, from mystical Christianity with the Centering Prayer, to Buddhist mindfulness meditation, the idea of attending to the present moment is more to do with allowing the dissolution of the ego (sense of separateness) by focussing on a sacred name or noble virtue. As with the repetition of a holy name or mantra advocated by Sathya Sai Baba, the Hari Krishnas and other groups originating in Asia, the Centering Prayer, resurrected from the Middle Ages by Father Thomas Keating, is a form of contemplation. Attention is focussed on the silent repetition of a sacred name (e.g. Jesus, Mother, Esu) or noble virtue (e.g. Silence, Calm, Love, Yes), while letting go of all thoughts (including sense perceptions, feelings, memories, and so on), so as to reconnect with our true Self, our

Oneness, our Peaceful Mind, Open Heart. There are many such forms of contemplative prayer in different traditions, requiring that we pause and participate in an intentional process of connecting with a state of mind or holy Presence outside of our day-to-day way of being.

As with the more secular mindfulness in recent times, prayer and religious affiliation in general have been demonstrated to be associated with increased longevity and well-being.

Psychologist Kenneth Pargament, in his 1997 book, *The Psychology of Religion*, reveals the research evidence for such rewards (and others) following on from being involved with what he refers to as an *integrated religion*, or the sincere practice of one's own form of spirituality.

Surprisingly, Pargament said that surveys investigating the extent of religiosity in the USA population found that 94 percent believe in God and 90 percent pray. Aside from the mounting body of research into the healing power of belief and placebo, it is also likely that those who pray (in whatever way) are growing additional networks of neurons similar to those triggered by the practice of modern-day mindfulness. It could be that our increasingly secular society is filling the vacuum left by the dramatic slide in church attendance in recent decades with the practice of mindfulness – climbing the same mountain as prayful and contemplative religion, but following a different pathway.

With the explosion of research into the effects of mindfulness on emotional wellbeing and mental health, work efficiency and learning in schools, there has been recognition of the need to define more carefully the common elements of the broad range of mindful awareness practices. Noting the connection that modern-day mindfulness techniques have with certain religious contemplative practices spanning the centuries, clinical psychologist

Scott Bishop and colleagues have proposed – for research purposes – that mindfulness can be seen as consisting of two main dimensions: the self-regulation of attention, and a certain orientation to experience.

In their 2002 publication, *Mindfulness: A Proposed Operational Definition,* they define these two dimensions as:

> *1. ... the self-regulation of attention so that it is maintained on immediate experience, thereby allowing for increased recognition of mental events in the present moment.*
> *2. ... a particular orientation toward one's experiences in the present moment, an orientation that is characterized by curiosity, openness, and acceptance.*

There are a number of self-report questionnaires on mindfulness, all having questions to be rated 'yes' or 'no', or 'not at all' up to 'much of the time'. Sample questions are in the nature of the following:

- ◇ I can be experiencing an emotion and not be aware of it until sometime later.
- ◇ I find it difficult to stay focussed on what is happening in the present.
- ◇ I tend to walk quickly to where I'm going without paying attention to what I experience along the way.
- ◇ I tend not to notice how tense I've become until later when it really grabs my attention.
- ◇ I am impatient with myself and with others.
- ◇ I rush through activities without much awareness of what I'm doing.
- ◇ I find myself preoccupied with the future or the past.
- ◇ I find myself doing things without paying attention.

Self-report questionnaires on mindfulness provide a reasonable before-and-after measure of how proficient we have become in being attentive to the present moment. An added benefit of answering the questions is that we feel motivated to change, after realising the extent to which we are moving through life as if 'asleep' (not being here, for the Now).

In a fairly recent attempt to find an operational definition of mindfulness, psychologist Ruth Baer and others were able to delineate five common themes appearing in recent scientific self-report questionnaires. As reported in their 2006 publication titled: *Using Self-Report Assessment Methods to Explore Facets of Mindfulness*, these five themes were:

1. Non-reactivity to inner experience (e.g. I perceive my feelings and emotions without having to react to them)
2. Observing/noticing/attending to sensations, perceptions, thoughts, feelings (e.g. I remain present with sensations and feelings even when they are unpleasant or painful)
3. Acting with awareness or concentration, without being distracted – that is, not on automatic pilot (e.g. I do not break or spill things because of carelessness, not paying attention, or thinking of something else)
4. Describing/labelling with words (e.g. I can easily put my beliefs, opinions, and expectations into words)
5. Non-judgmental of experience (e.g. I do not tell myself I shouldn't be thinking the way I'm thinking)

The psychiatrist Daniel Siegel uses the acronym of *COAL* to help his patients understand how to practise mindfulness. That is, we engage in our here-and-now experience with **C**uriosity, **O**penness, **A**cceptance and **L**ove.

This Love is Love for ourself, for our breath, for the perfection underlying the exquisite order that arranges everything that we are noticing.

Some will wonder if we really can cultivate such Love for ourselves? Research into mindful awareness indicates that we can. Approaching mindfulness as a form of relationship with ourself allows us to see how this can be accomplished. When we regard mindfulness as a form of intrapersonal attunement, we come closer to seeing how we can become our own best friend through the practice of mindfulness. The question to ask ourselves is this: Would we treat our best friend with kindness or hostility? That is, we need to relate with kindness, with love, to all aspects of ourselves that we are noticing in each unfolding moment, whether it be our breath, our getting distracted, an unpleasant emotion, a hostile thought, in fact, all of our poignant human condition with all of its highs and lows, darkness and light. In other words, we are attuning to our higher Self who regards all and everything from the mountain top of pure Love.

Such attunement is at the heart of all caring relationships, whether between parent and child, teacher and student, therapist and patient/client, friends, and close colleagues. Along with others like Daniel Siegel, we are proposing that, in relating to others with mindful awareness, the mind enters a state of being in which one's here-and-now experiences are sensed directly, accepted for what they are, and acknowledged with kindness and respect. This is the kind of interpersonal attunement that promotes Love. And when the same level of kindness and respect is present in our being mindfully aware of (and attuned to) ourself, Love is there – Love for ourself, for this little self that so yearns to unite with our true Self, with the vast, limitless ocean of Love that we truly are.

Cultivating Mindfulness

In his 1990 book, *Full Catastrophe Living*, Jon Kabat-Zinn recommends seven attitudinal requirements for gaining the most from any practice of mindfulness. These are:

- Non-judging
- Patience

- ❖ Beginner's mind (experiencing things as if for the first time)
- ❖ Trust
- ❖ Non-striving
- ❖ Acceptance
- ❖ Letting go

Non-judging

Focussing on the here and now is not judging whether this is good or bad, better or worse than what we've known before, or what we had hoped for. It means adopting the stance of the impartial witness to our thoughts, feelings, sensations and experiences. Being mindful requires us to just be aware of whatever we are observing, without trying to label it or change it. One analogy is that of the baby in the cot who smiles upon seeing a thief come into the room – no judging, no concept of whether this is a virtuous or wicked person.

Patience

If we are feeling impatient, we are not being mindful, not being aware of the present moment, but rather wishing for some future event. When we are being patient, we know that the experience unfolding before our eye of awareness has its own perfect timing. Wishing that this moment will soon pass so that we can enjoy the next is like hoping that a blooming flower on a bush will soon fade so that we can enjoy the next one to appear.

Beginner's Mind

Having a beginner's mind when practising mindfulness is not something new for any of us – it is just that we've forgotten. When we were babies, we were totally open, seeing everything as if for the very first time, rejoicing in what we were finding anew in this present moment. If we can allow ourselves to feel as if we are born with the dawn of each new day, with each new second, we will be able to reclaim our beginner's mind. It takes practice, but even one sip of the ocean gives us a taste of the never-ending expanse of beauty and perfection we are immersed in. Cultivating the mind in this way enriches our relationship with ourselves, our family and every familiar part of our lives.

Trust

In the practice of mindfulness we can trust that, in the same way that we were guided from deep within ourselves in learning to walk, so too that same intuitive sense of direction is always there, regardless of mistakes along the way. We learn to trust that we are not our body, thoughts and feelings; but rather we are the resident in the body, the unchanging Witness who is observing all of this. We trust that every thought, feeling and sensation that we observe is perfect; it has a purpose in the great scheme of things. We can trust that whatever another person says or does to us, and whatever calamity or boon is presented to us, it will be perfect for our personal growth and learning.

Non-striving

Mindfulness has no goal other than for us to just be ourselves. There are no 'shoulds' in non-striving, only the commitment to do everything when necessary, with 100 percent of our energy and ability. A tiny ant struggling to drag along a leaf that is 30 times its size and weight, although obviously giving the task all that it has, is not caught up in the striving that we wish to avoid in mindfulness.

And the sun is not striving when it sacrifices so much of itself to heat and illuminate our world – if it did strive to burn more intensely, life would soon cease to exist on Earth. That is, the key to non-striving is to not try too hard, but rather, taking whatever action is needed, immersing ourselves fully in the activity.

When we are living mindfully, we are not trying to swim against the current

– we are going with the flow of the moment-to-moment experience, sometimes fast, at other times slow, but always towards, and not away from, our certain destiny of becoming one with the Ocean within that awaits us, our higher Self.

Acceptance

Living mindfully has much to do with accepting things as they are, ourselves included. Acceptance means: not denying what is there in front of us; making room for our feelings instead of trying to push them away; recognising that all types of thoughts can enter our mind, each one offering a choice as to which pathway to follow; and understanding that other people are merely playing the role that has been assigned to them in this drama of life. We fully accept that the blind man can't see, not expecting otherwise. Yet acceptance is not a passive resignation about our blind spots, our character failings. We can accept that we have an unwanted habit, accept that we might rid ourselves of it in a day or several years, and accept that we are stumbling about in the dark looking for an antidote. In most situations, careful attention paid to every link in the sequence of happenings that make up a habit will be sufficient to weaken and abolish it.

Letting go

In the practice of mindfulness, the opposite of letting go is 'holding' – holding on to an attitude, judgment, thought, feeling, sensation, and so on. Letting go, in mindfulness, is the same as when Christians say, "I let go and let God." If we cannot let go of something that the mind is holding on to, we can observe the 'holding' from the vantage point of an impartial, non-judgmental, compassionate observer. Letting go is like putting down two suitcases full of old rubbish; it is the letting go of fixed ideas about how we, or the world, should be or behave.

The quality of our mindfulness will be affected by the extent to which we can abide by these seven requirements for giving unfettered attention to something, moment to moment. It is not something that we can just decide to do. Our mental/emotional habits, attitudes, likes and dislikes have well-established networks of neuronal activity in the brain. It will require diligent practice in our everyday lives if we are to neutralize these customary ways of thinking that limit our perception.

The Universality of the Breath in Mindfulness Practices

Most of the research studies with both adults and children have used the breath as the focal point on which to centre the mind's attention. This could be because the breath has some important features that aid in the practice of mindfulness. For example, our breath is always with us, and its rhythmic nature – like the endless rising and falling of the waves in the ocean – automatically brings calm to the nervous system when attention is directed there. Also the breath is the interface between the internal and the external, the voluntary and the involuntary, the automatic and the effortful – these features might play a part in how focussing attention on the breath can bring increased clarity and peace of mind, and an opening of the heart.

A typical guided mindfulness practice using a breath-focus would begin something like this:

> *Make yourself comfortable. Close the eyes ... Now bring your attention to your breathing ... observing the breath ... As thoughts come, just let them go, and return your attention to your breathing ...*
> *Follow the air as it comes in through your nostrils and goes down to the bottom of your lungs ... then follow it as it goes back out again ... Keep letting go of thinking, and keep returning your attention to the breath ... Notice the air moving in and out of your nostrils ... Notice how it's slightly warmer as it comes out, and cooler as it goes in ...*

The Benefits of Mindfulness

With the development of modern biomedical technology, researchers have been able to demonstrate in a wide range of studies that the practice of mindfulness, even for thirty minutes every day, has a helpful effect on the body, mind and emotions. The range of beneficial effects in adults brought about by even a short course of five to ten hours in breath-focussed mindfulness includes:

- Reduction in stress levels
- Lessening the impact of chronic physical pain
- Boosting the body's immune system
- Improved attention and concentration
- Enhancing the full range of positive emotions
- Reducing addictive behaviours
- Enhancing performance in work, sport or academics
- Stimulating and releasing creativity
- Increased interpersonal skills
- Improved control over strong negative emotions like anger, fear and greed
- Coping with painful life events, such as death of a loved one

That the practice of mindfulness can have such a wide-ranging positive effect upon the social, cognitive, emotional and physical wellbeing of people suggests that it is one way in which the brain turns its focus inwardly to promote balance and harmony.

Buddhists and meditators from other disciplines have been using such focussed-attention techniques for thousands of hours and, through diligent practice, have been able to attest from their own experience that it is a worthwhile form of self -discipline for every human being – that is, its value is universal and does not require allegiance to a particular Faith or religious dogma. Further, Buddhist monks who have practised mindful meditation intensively over several years have measurably different brain structures in the pre-frontal cortex, allowing them to go into a deep inner quietude within just a few seconds.

We live in a time when developments in neuroscience are rapidly beginning to provide neurobiological explanations as to why the practice of mindfulness has such beneficial effects. Daniel Siegel, co-director of the UCLA Mindful Awareness Research Centre and author of *The Mindful Brain*, shares the research consensus that mindful awareness practices fall into the category of self-directed neural plasticity exercises – that is, they change the actual function and structure of the brain. When self-discipline is called upon to shift attention away from the more entrenched, habitual patterns of neural firing, and cultivate the growth of new specialised brain cells that form linkages to thousands of other neurons, we can be confident of building a pathway to wholeness and wellbeing. The abandoned cells gradually die off and the new ones receiving attention multiply, thereby replacing old habits of thinking, feeling and behaving with the new more desirable ones. As Dan Siegel says, "Where attention goes, neural firing occurs. And where neurons fire, new connections can be made." With sustained practice in focussed attention, a more flexible way of responding to the world develops, giving us the freedom to make choices denied to us previously.

Living mindfully is really about being alive, alive in the sense of benefitting from these few decades we have been granted to live in a body that was once very young, then matured, and now, whether we are 20 or 80, is advancing inexorably towards its closing years.

Some refer to our being born into the University of Life. We know that, if we were to sleep throughout every lecture in the subjects we've enrolled in at college, the chances of gaining our sought-after reward at the end would be minimal or non-existent. In the same way, we are all enrolled in this life to learn the metaphysics of Peaceful Mind, Open Heart – to rediscover our true Self, manifesting as the Human Values of Love, Truth, Peace, Right Conduct and Non-violence. The diligent practice of mindful awareness, of being awake to the richness of each moment-to-moment experience, ensures that we will pass all of our examinations. We will find inner peace in potentially stressful situations; recognise beauty and harmony amidst chaos and confusion; realise that who we really are is exquisite and extraordinary; and rediscover again and again that pure Love and perfection permeate everything and everybody, even what appears to be their opposite.

Be yourself. Life is precious as it is.
All the elements for your happiness are already here.
There is no need to run, strive, search or struggle.
Just be.

Thich Nhat Hanh

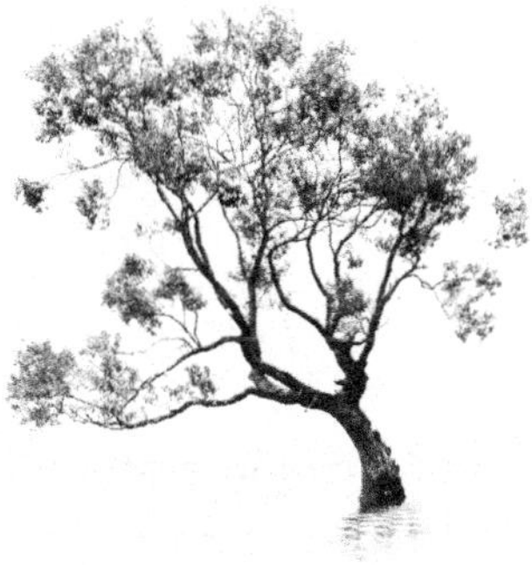

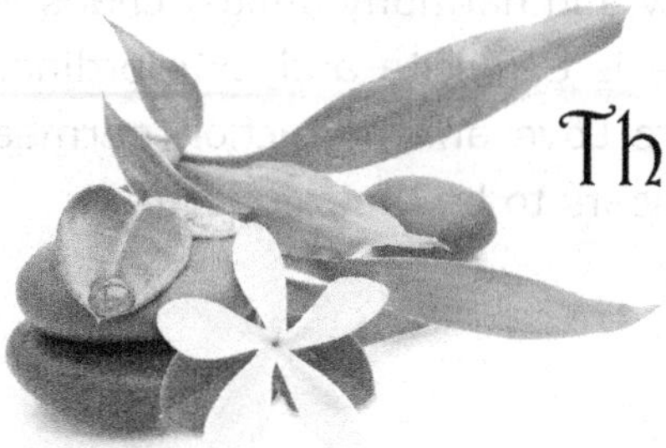

The Practice

EXERCISES FOR MINDFUL AWARENESS

As noted in earlier chapters, we need self-awareness before we can engage in self-regulation. Applying this to mindfulness, we can begin by assessing ourselves on how well we are living in the present moment, in the Now, with non-judgmental acceptance of ourself and others. With this information, we are in a strong position to change the way we live in the world, rediscovering the peace, love, beauty and joy that come with enhanced mindful awareness.

<u>Exercise 1:</u>
How Can I Be More Mindful?

How can I do this exercise?

- ◇ Please rate each of the following statements using the scale provided. Write the number that best describes your own opinion of what is generally true for you.

1	2	3	4
Rarely	Occasionally	Fairly Often	Almost Always

1. I am open to the experience of the present moment.

2. I sense my body, whether eating, cooking, cleaning or talking.
3. When I notice that my mind has been wandering, I gently return to the experience of the here and now.
4. I am able to appreciate myself.
5. I pay attention to what's behind my actions.
6. I see my mistakes and difficulties without judging them.
7. I feel connected to my experience in the here-and-now.
8. I accept unpleasant experiences.
9. I am friendly to myself when things go wrong.
10. I watch my feelings without getting lost in them.
11. In difficult situations, I can pause without immediately reacting.
12. I experience moments of inner peace and ease, even when things get hectic and stressful.
13. I am patient with myself and with others.
14. I am able to smile when I notice how I sometimes make life difficult.

______Summary Score

◇ Select one of the mindfulness statements with the lowest rating.

◇ Endeavour to pay attention to this aspect of being mindful, as often as you can, for a whole day; then, select another low-scored one to focus on for the next day; and so on.

◇ Use the questionnaire to assess your level of mindfulness again, one month from now; and thereafter every month.

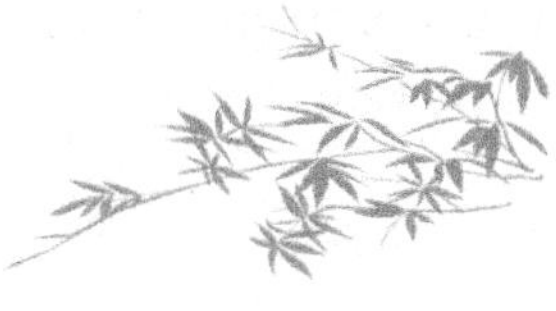

Exercise 2:

Mindfulness in Everyday Activities

How can I do this exercise?

◇ Re-read and reflect on the seven pillars of mindfulness (non-judging, patience, beginner's mind, trust, non-striving, acceptance, letting go) described earlier in this chapter.

◇ Select just one of these (e.g. beginner's mind) for practice in an everyday activity.

◇ Choose one activity that you engage in daily (e.g. eating, showering, dressing, any walking, listening, and so on).

◇ Each time you are engaged in this activity, ask yourself, "Am I doing this mindfully? Am I doing this with (for example) a beginner's mind, noticing everything as if for the first time?"

◇ After you have focussed on this one pillar of mindfulness (e.g. beginner's mind) for one week or so, select another pillar (e.g. non-judging) to focus on.

◇ Select the same or a different activity and repeat the above process. That is, "Am I doing this mindfully? Am I doing this with (for example) an attitude of non-judging?"

◇ If you find this exercise interesting and beneficial, you might like to do it for each one of the seven pillars of mindfulness, for a number of different everyday activities.

Exercise 3:
Mindfulness of Breathing

The breath is always with us, and so it is a reliable post to which we can tether our wandering mind. At any time of the day, in any situation, we can bring our attention to our breath, even for a few seconds.

This present exercise will help you to become familiar with being mindful of the breath. You might like to practise at first by reading it aloud to a friend (slowly, following the pause times), asking them to follow. After a few practices with other people, you'll find it easy for you to do it for yourself without having to read the instructions.

How can I do this exercise?

- ◇ Sit with your back straight ... (2 sec.), feet flat on the floor ... (2 sec.), hands resting on your thighs or in your lap ... (2 sec.). Bend the head slightly down ... (2 sec.), eyes closed ... (2 sec.) or half-close the eyes and look at one spot on the floor ... (5 sec.).

- ◇ Bring your attention to your breathing ... (5 sec.).

- ◇ Follow the air as it comes in through your nostrils and goes down to the bottom of your lungs ... (2 sec.), then follow it as it goes back out again ... (5 sec.).

- ◇ Notice the air moving in and out of your nostrils ... (3 sec.). Notice how it's slightly warmer as it comes out, and cooler as it goes in ... (10 sec.).

- ◇ Notice the gentle rise and fall of your rib cage ... (2 sec.), as you breathe ... (10 sec.).

◇ Notice the gentle rise and fall of your belly ... (2 sec.), as you breathe ... (10 sec.).

◇ Fix your attention on one of these areas, whichever you prefer: on the breath at the nostrils ... (2 sec.), on the breath in the ribcage ... (2 sec.) or the breath in the belly ... (5 sec.).

◇ Keep your attention on this part of the body ... (2 sec.), noticing the movement in and out of the breath ... (10 sec.).

◇ Allow any feelings to come and go as they please ... (2 sec.), whether pleasant or unpleasant ... (5 sec.), and keep returning your attention to the breath ... (10 sec.).

◇ Thoughts will come ... (2 sec.), sometimes pleasant ... (2 sec.), sometimes unpleasant ... (2 sec.). Allow them to come, and then let them go ... (5 sec.) and keep returning your attention to the breath ... (10 sec.).

◇ It doesn't matter how often the mind wanders off ... (2 sec.). Each time it wanders..(1 sec.), just let go of the thought ... (2 sec.), and bring your attention back to the breath ... (10 sec.). Keep returning your attention to the breath ... (5 sec.). This is mindful breathing ... (20 to 30 sec.).

◇ When you are ready ... (1 sec.), bring yourself back to the room ... (2 sec.). Wiggle your hands and feet ... (2 sec.) and open your eyes.

Exercise 4:

Brief Mindfulness Exercise

This short exercise is ideal for taking a short break away from a challenging work situation, or when you are feeling a little stressed.

How can I do this exercise?

- ◇ Notice three things you can see (e.g. pen, chair, etc.). Calmly look at each one for 5 seconds.
- ◇ Notice three things you can hear (e.g. talking, car sounds, etc.). Focus on each sound for about 5 seconds.
- ◇ Notice three things your body is touching (e.g. clothes, chair, etc.). Keep your attention on each one for about 5 seconds.

Realize deeply that the present moment is all you ever have.
Make the Now the primary focus of your life.

Eckhart Tolle

Chapter 12

Living in the Present Moment

You must live in the present, launch yourself on every wave,
find your eternity in each moment.

Henry David Thoreau

There is a story of a man who was just beginning to get grey hair and lose some of the power of his legs. This made him wary about becoming old, with fearful thoughts about frailty and infirmity. He sought out the wise one who lived in the forest and asked, "Holy One, is there anything I can do to ensure that I am peaceful and happy in my closing years?" The Holy One answered, "As little as you can do to make the sun rise in the morning." "Then of what use," the surprised seeker asked, "are these mindfulness exercises that you prescribe?" "To make sure," the elder said, "that you are not asleep when the sun begins to rise."

When we are attending to the present moment – whether focussing on the caress of our life-giving breath, attuning to another, or listening to the 'sound of the universe' underneath all of the sounds reaching our ears, a special kind of happiness and contentment arrives like a sudden breeze through an open window. So unexpected, delighting us with its presence, even when the visit is for just a few seconds, the warm glow and sense of upliftment stay with us like a fragrance in the air long after the wave of bliss moves on.

Such inner delight does not have the familiarity of those earth-bound pleasures that are dependent upon the satisfaction of the ego and the senses; rather, it has an air of mystery about it, hinting at a vast unknown of beauty as yet to be made manifest within us. But, at the same time, this one jewel of the Treasure feels like it belongs to us somehow, as if we are kindred spirits. It is like coming Home for a while, feeling the warmth of the fire in the hearth. Somehow we don't feel exultation at having found something so precious – it is more a sense of gratitude that our higher Self has finally gained our attention.

How blessed we are to know that 'a vast, limitless ocean of nectar divine' lies waiting within, calling us to the centre of ourselves. Such a blessing to know that the Treasure we are seeking is all the while seeking us, prompting us to become mindfully aware of the jewels that are scattered around our feet.

Because the Holy Grail is hidden within us, in a place where few would look, the tendency to dwell in the past as we get older becomes more enticing. With less to occupy our days, and less of a future to anticipate, we can fill our minds with nostalgic recollections, sometimes with fondness, and at other times with remorse, resentment, longing or sadness.

When we pore back over the years in this way, we put on dark glasses that deny us from seeing the sunshine here now in our lives; we weigh ourselves down with old bags from the past that are of no use for the journey we are now on. And we flirt with the error of delusion, for the past is not real. It is but a dream, like a mirage in the desert that will keep us from finding the water to keep us alive.

It is not that the past is of no value – all dreams have wisdom to offer. If we can recall the images and feelings from the past and examine them again with the eyes of the healer, the alchemist, the Wise One, then base metal can be transmuted into gold. What was once so delightful will be seen as a mirror showing untold wealth inside; the regret over past decisions will be viewed as the perfect turning of the river as it heads towards the open sea; and the anger towards those who wronged us will change to a compassion for their being so blind. Re-running the movie of our life in this way – triumphs and tragedies both – rather than engaging in nostalgic reminiscence or resentful recrimination, we allow the possibility of being nourished by the inner meaning and purpose of the events in our life.

When we do look back – or, rather, bring the past into our present awareness with conscious intent – it helps to re-experience each scene from the past with a beginner's mind, even if we have already replayed the same movie many times before. The other six pillars of mindfulness (non-judging, patience, trust, letting go, acceptance and non-striving) are also of value in this replaying the movie of the past in our mind – particularly *letting go* – as will be seen as we proceed.

The work of releasing the past is not easy, especially when our minds are preoccupied with unfinished business. It is a paradox of mindful living that, without having embraced our past, we cannot let it go; or, as a sage once said, "We cannot transform what we have not first blessed."

But, how to bless? How can we reflect back on a painful event with sufficient acceptance, non-judgment, trust and forgiveness so as to be able to feel a sense of gratitude that it happened? It sounds impossible, particularly for those dark abuses which left us, even years later, wondering if life was worth living anymore. And yet, little by little, like the wearing away of stone by the steady drip of gentle water, the wounds can be healed, eventually to such an extent that we can say, "When the lightning bolt struck the tree, devastation was wrought, but thereafter came green shoots for a new forest in the making. Once I was that tree; now I am this veritable forest, vibrating and dancing with life."

As noted in an earlier chapter, Baba Ram Dass, a former Harvard university professor in psychology, had influenced the spiritual lives of a generation through his 1971 book on mindful living, *Be Here Now*. After decades of being an inspirational force in this field, he suffered a massive stroke. By the year 2000, Ram Dass had sufficiently recovered to write another book, *Still Here : Embracing Aging, Changing and Dying*, from the standpoint of a veteran teacher who was now applying the principles of mindfulness to his present situation (growing old, being severely incapacitated). On the benefits of bringing a focussed attention to recollection of the past he wrote:

> *There's a great difference between wallowing in the past, turning each detail over endlessly in one's mind until one is stuck there, and 'experiencing' it with one's present consciousness ... By embracing the past into the present, our minds are able to enter a kind of choiceless awareness in which past experience can float up and pass away, with no clinging or judgment. When we do that, the memories get 'neutralized'; they become part of the backdrop of existence, and the energy that has been locked into holding onto the past is released. We feel a little freer, a little more alive.*

The term *choiceless awareness* used in the above quote brings a different perspective on how to view both the past and the present. We wrote earlier about the analogy of the movie screen – the images of life are projected onto the screen of awareness. We are the screen not the movie.

The screen (our higher Self) is *aware* of the images (present events and memories of the past) being projected onto it, yet it is not exercising a *choice* to be aware – it is always aware. That is, our Soul or higher Self (the screen) is in a perpetual state of choiceless awareness, ready for us to observe our life (and the past) from the standpoint of being this eternal Witness.

Re-running the movie of the past while in a state of mindful (choiceless) awareness creates what Ram Dass calls a *wisdom barrier*. That is, we are viewing the past from the standpoint of our Soul, the higher Self, the wisdom Self. Our innate wisdom allows us to confront painful or traumatic events, or the deep regret at having taken a wrong path in life, without becoming stuck in resentment or self-pity. For example, we might decide to remain mindfully aware of our breath (watching it every moment) while we look at past events. In this way we are bringing the past into the present moment, and it is viewed in a different light. The past is compelled to release its hold on us, and we feel a shift away from these old attachments.

Once we learn to look at the past through the eyes of the present, what we discover is the degree to which our thoughts and feelings have been frozen in time. Although we may have changed tremendously with age, we have carried with us the interpretation, and emotional effect, of past events as they occurred then. This has been making us feel fragmented, incomplete, as if we've been missing out on something, something that would bring closure, allowing us to sense the perfect order and meaning running through our lives like a golden chord linking all the precious beads into a priceless necklace. Re-experiencing these memories and feelings from the Soul's perspective allows the necklace to reveal itself.

All of us can remember moments in our lives when we did step into observing life from our Soul's perspective, when we were oblivious to all except being in this ongoing, moment-to-moment Now. These sojourns in our Treasure House, in the state of Peaceful Mind and Open Heart, stand out as different from other memories we carry. They are mirrors, presented to us so we can catch a glimpse of who we really are.

In so many ways, our memories of the past distract us from living in the here and now. They can be like weeds in the garden, leaving little room for the flowers to grow. As we cultivate an ability to be more and more deeply in the moment, the power of the moment becomes stronger than the memories of the past – even memories of extreme pain.

When we plant enough flowers to fill up the whole garden, there is no room left for the weeds to grow. Every second of being mindful of this present moment, every time we look at something in the past with the eyes of the Soul, the ever-present Witness, our sense of who we are expands a step further into greater and greater spaciousness; and, in turn, as we move closer to identifying with our higher Self, so too does the beauty, wonder and exquisiteness of the present moment reveal itself.

Shedding Attachment to the Future

The present is the product of the past and the future is the result of the present. If we planted corn a few months ago, it will be corn that we are reaping today; if it is soybeans we are planting today, surely it will be soybeans that we will harvest in the future. That is, both the past and the future are present in what *is*, because it is the fruit of the past and the seed of the future. It makes sense, therefore, to live in the present – with mindful awareness of the here-and-now: entertaining good thoughts; nurturing good feelings and doing good deeds without selfish motive; extending love and compassion towards all beings. Having planted the right seeds, we can be confident of seeing them harvested sometime in the future – in this way we can let go of concern and worry for whatever the future holds. If at some stage in the past we have planted the seeds of selfishness and ill will, it is understandable that they too will be presenting their fruits sometime in the future. Since we cannot undo what has been done by us in the past, it is only appropriate that we should accept the future consequences of whatever thoughts, words and actions we may have planted, without demur.

With this reasoning always there to remind us to come into the present moment, as we do so we not only discover that we're able to free ourselves from the past, but from the future as well. As the Tibetan teaching instructs, we learn not to invite the future into our thoughts before its time, thereby shielding ourselves from unnecessary discomfort; for, just as the past traps us in memories, the future traps us in anticipation which so often can lead to disappointment. As Baba Ram Dass has said:

> *Confronted by daunting challenges and expectations, many older people spend a great deal of their lives dreading what lies ahead. Although death is certainly our greatest fear, we also preoccupy ourselves with other concerns that take us away from our current experience and cast us into the sea of what-ifs. This is a futile enterprise; although we must plan for our future by putting our affairs in order, there is nothing to be gained through the sort of obsessive worrying and fretful expectation that characterizes the thinking of many older people.*

Most of our fears, if we look at them clearly, relate to how we imagine the future will be. Fear thrives on the unknown, and although many of us avoid what scares us, it is more effective to approach our fears as closely as possible – to bring our ideas of the future into the present.

In 1987, Susan Jeffers published her book, *Feel the Fear and Do it Anyway,* which has proved to be widely popular, essentially because its title gives the simple means for dealing with fear. Several hundred years earlier, the Sufi spiritual order reminded us that: 'Fear is the door to the unknown. Unbolt that door'. And, more recently, the esoteric Christianity teaching guide, *A Course in Miracles*, tells us that: 'There are only two emotions, Love and fear. And fear is but the shadow of Love'. That is, the fear-shadow appears when the light of our Love is blocked.

To dissolve all of our worries and fears about how much we might suffer as we move into old age, the method is to bring each one of our apprehensions, one by one over time, into the present moment, with love and compassion. To use mindful breathing again as an example, one approach is to spend a few minutes focussing on the breath in the centre of the chest, imagining that we are breathing in pure Love. Then we imagine one of our concerns, visualising it happening, while continuing to focus on the breath filled with love and compassion. As we do this, feeding the Love much more than the fear, the latter will lose its intensity. That is, feel the fear and do it anyway, with Love. Love is the antidote for all fear, and every present moment is full of Love, for Love is all there is.

Time and Change

We all know that time is eternal; it has no end; it is boundless. In an esoteric sense, time does not change, for it is always present. What does change is our concept of time. Time and change are interrelated. We measure time by what changes, and we measure change in increments of time. For many of us, when we have anxiety about what might befall us as we grow old, it's really because we fear change. Change means uncertainty, and many types of uncertainty create fear.

Of course, there are occasions when people enjoy uncertainty (e.g. betting), but it's when our ego – the concept we have of ourself – is confronted with the possibility of its having to change, then we have fear. That is, the thought of becoming incontinent and unable to recognise those we love, is fearful because our ego sees itself as becoming severely limited and damaged.

Our ego is our concept of who we are. Generally, we believe that we are this body, this personality, this brain and these common human abilities to converse, remember, make decisions, control our feelings and so on. Naturally, our ego fears its own destruction.

To deal with this uncertainty of change, with the possibility of degeneration of mind and body, we have to begin letting go of believing that we are all of these things that change. We need to identify more with that Essence within us that does not change. We need to identify with the One who is observing all of this change, the ever-present Witness, our higher Self, our eternal Soul or Spirit. Along with Baba Ram Dass and so many others, we refer to this approach to growing old as *conscious aging*; that is, by remaining ever-conscious of the present moment, our timelessness, we can observe with dispassion all that is changing with time (our thoughts, feelings, breath, sounds, etc.).

Recognising that we are *not* this body and mind that are aging, while at the same time having the very compelling experience that we *are* this body/mind complex, seems to be paradoxical. To paraphrase the words of the holy ones, "We are eternal beings having a time-bound human experience." Or, to use the language of nuclear physics, "We are all waves of energy on the one vast, limitless ocean of energy." Accepting and being comfortable with paradox is the key to finding our Peaceful Mind, Open Heart as each breath takes us further along the path of aging.

This is where our conscious aging can help to relieve the anxiety we feel over change. While the ever-present Witness, our higher Self, knows only the eternity of time, our ego self sees the seconds ticking by. By learning to remain in both time perspectives, we experience a stillness that enables us to accept the turbulence of change. Becoming free of the ego's wanting things to remain as they are, and becoming more familiar with what exists eternally within ourselves in every moment, we gradually arrive at approaching change with curiosity instead of dread, and at being more comfortable with 'not knowing' than we have been before.

One of the unsettling things about the changes that come with aging is how our images of ourselves contradict the reality. However much we might still feel young, our bodies invariably tell us otherwise. The older we get, the more likely we are to experience these moments when self-image and reality contradict each other. Though this experience is disturbing, it gives us information about what we need to let go of, and where we need to pay attention. Just as physical pain alerts us to troubles in the body, mental pain tells us where we need to be more conscious. In other words, our anxiety, sadness, delusions, and so on can become our greatest helpers in freeing ourselves from suffering. They point to where the ego is trapped, and remind us to begin shifting our identity to the Soul level, to where we are resisting change, to the level of the higher Self. Ram Dass says:

> *Our curriculum of conscious aging requires that we get as close as possible with the thing that's scaring us, in order to reveal our attachments, and to experience the serenity that comes with letting go of them.*

The European mystic of the 1930's in France, G. I. Gurdjieff, urged his students to engage in what he called *conscious suffering* which involves the same principle as that for conscious aging – that is, to consciously go in the direction of our discomforts and fears so as to awaken from our habitual or programmed way of living in the world. It rests on the assumption that each one of our apprehensions about illness, aging and dying is pointing to a compost heap of outdated thinking that can be used to grow new flowers of self-assurance, wisdom and fearlessness in the garden of our aging years.

By confronting ourselves consciously and deliberately with the changes that worry or frighten us, we learn to weaken our dread of the future. Having seen the inevitability of change, we are not surprised or overwhelmed when the laws of Nature take their course. This does not do away with pain but it does cast a different light upon suffering, so that we can shoulder our burdens with more dignity and good nature, having prepared ourselves for these changes.

In the end, of course, our approach to the future comes down to how we feel about mystery. As much as we may know of ourselves and our existence, there will always be a great deal more that we will never know.

Even though we know that what happens in our future has already been determined according to what seeds of thoughts, words and deeds we have planted in the past, the events that will unfold are essentially a mystery. Our challenge is to love the mystery, in the same way that the flute has no way of knowing what note will be played through it by the musician in the next moment. Our future as we age is not known, but we can trust that whatever life presents to us is what we are ready for. We are greater than what we think we are, with vast inner reservoirs of each one of the five Human Values of Love, Truth, Peace, Right Conduct and Non-violence waiting to be tapped into as sustenance for our journey.

The Timeless Present

When we want to go for a walk, we get ready by putting on our shoes. When we are to travel overnight somewhere, we pack our clothes in a bag. But what preparations are we making for the journey through our closing years, and for the ultimate journey, our departure from this body?

Both journeys are inevitable and are a part of this great journey of life that we are engaged in. Instead of preparing ourselves for these end-parts of the adventure, there is often anxiety and lamentations – these only serve to distract us from the reality that the deserts, valleys and mountains that we travel through are rich in colour and harmony. So, how are we to prepare? How are we to make ready for the possibility of having to deal with any one of the many possible physical and mental ailments that can accompany aging, or for those last hours and days before our final breath exhales?

The answer to our question lies in the present moment, for, as has often been said, there is no time in this moment, this Now. When our attention is fully engaged in the present moment, we lose track of time. With our mind no longer blinkered and limited by old time-bound habits of comparing 'this' to what used to be or judging 'that' to be good or bad – all of which relate to memories of the past or hopes and expectations for the future – we are free to discover the hidden grandeur and beauty in everyday experiences.

By developing the habit of 'being here now', of mindful awareness, with singular focus on the here-and-now, the landscape and surroundings will remain delightful and enriching even as we move into the latter part of our journey through life. We discover that what we have to offer to the world is not limited by the passing years, nor by the condition of our mind and bodies. Let us share with you an inspiring example of treasuring the *what is*, that which is most holy. Our story concerns a very high Lama in Tibet who had written to the 13th Dalai Lama sometime around 1900 lamenting how, now that he was blind, almost deaf, crippled and incontinent, a great darkness had come upon him because he could no longer be of any use to his many thousands of followers. In his wisdom, the 13th Dalai Lama wrote back something to the effect of:

> *You might well believe that you can no longer be of loving service to those in your jurisdiction, but this is a transparently false assumption. Let me assure you that you can now be of even greater service than ever before, for now you have the opportunity to feel compassion, real compassion. Now you know what it feels like to be rendered useless in the eyes of society, what it is like to lose even more of your dignity and self-confidence as your health declines still further. You do not have to go anywhere or even be with anyone to do your good work. From this moment on, your compassion and loving kindness will radiate out from you as a constant stream of healing energy to all those who are suffering with being blind, deaf, crippled and incontinent, in fact to all beings throughout the world who are sunk in despair and self-pity. The loving service so rendered is beyond compare.*

The effect on the high Lama upon reading these words was powerful and immediate. He spent the rest of his days in quiet, contented seclusion, beaming out his love and compassion to the whole world. To our understanding, he was able to respond so readily to the timely advice from his great mentor because he was already well-practised in living in the moment, treasuring the perfection of what is happening right now, and so was able to find a deep meaning and purpose in his debilitated condition – he just needed to be reminded.

We too can begin to develop this skill of living in the timeless present, simply by learning to give our full attention to one thing at a time. That is, when we are drinking tea, drink tea. When we are washing the dishes, wash the dishes. We can say to ourselves, with each new move, "Now I am raising the cup to my lips. Now I can smell the aroma and feel the hot tea upon my lips," and so on. This helps to slow the mind as it ceases to run after the future or hark back to the past. When we attend, with care, to our present activity, we discover a wonderful freedom from our incessant thoughts. In the next step, the next turning on of the water tap, in the next breath, no time exists. Whenever we take the opportunity to come fully into the present moment, we catch a glimpse of how wonderful it is to rest in the eternal present.

To see a world in a grain of sand and a heaven in a wild flower,
hold infinity in the palm of your hand and
eternity in an hour.

William Blake

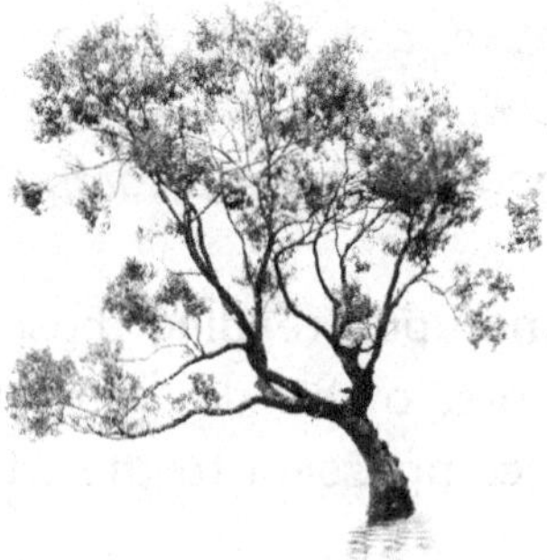

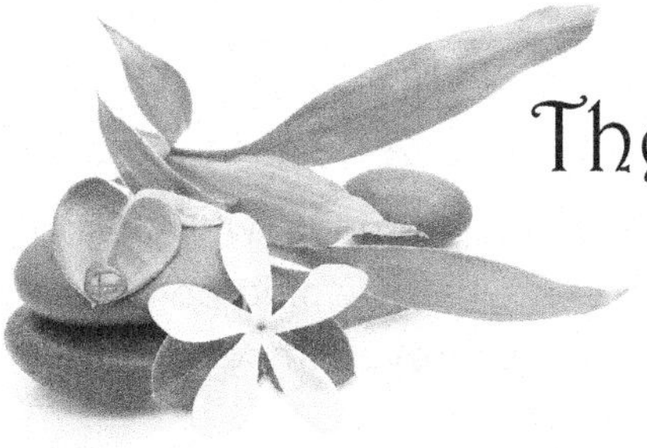

The Practice

EXERCISES FOR LIVING MINDFULLY

If we want to be happy when we are elderly we must begin practising that art in these our earlier years. Happiness arises from within, at those times when we are in touch with our true Self, in the present moment.

To practise mindfulness (choiceless awareness or focussed attention), certain attitudes of mind are required. These are: non-judging, patience, beginner's mind, trust, non-striving, acceptance, letting go. Each one ensures that we remain focussed on what is being noticed in the present moment, without being distracted by thoughts of the future or reminiscences of the past. As was outlined in earlier pages, each one of the seven pillars of mindfulness can be used as a check on the quality of our mindful awareness – if the opposite of any one of them is present, it's an indication that we are caught up in either the future or the past in one way of another.

The exercises to follow are to give us practice in being mindful, while keeping in mind just one of these seven pillars of mindfulness.

<u>Exercise 1:</u>
Living Mindfully with Acceptance

How can I do this exercise?

◇ Return to Chapter 11 and read through again the description given for living with an attitude of *Acceptance*.

◇ Find a quiet time and place.

◇ Spend a few minutes reading through the poem below, reflecting on each line, imagining as well as you can what it would be like to live each moment with full *Acceptance* of whatever images come into your mind.

> Allow your life to unfold naturally.
> Know that it too is a vessel of perfection.
> Just as you breathe in and breathe out,
> there is a time for being ahead
> and a time for being behind;
> a time for being in motion
> and a time for being at rest;
> a time for being vigorous
> and a time for being exhausted;
> a time for being safe
> and a time for being in danger.
> To the sage, all of life is a movement towards perfection.

◇ Think of someone in your life to practise with, in imagination. It could be a friend, family member, client, stranger or work colleague.

◇ Imagine that you are in the presence of that person, practising being totally *accepting* of them – for one day, one week, one month, one year.

Exercise 2:
Living Mindfully without Judgment

How can I do this exercise?

◇ Return to Chapter 11 and read through again the description given there for living with an attitude of *Non-judging*.

◇ Find a quiet time and place.

◇ Spend a few minutes reading through the poem below, reflecting on each line, imagining as best you can what it would be like to live each moment being totally *non-judging* of whatever images come into your mind.

> The sage has no fixed mind;
> he is aware of the needs of others.
> Those who are good he treats with goodness.
> Those who are bad he also treats with goodness,
> because the nature of his being is good.

◇ Think of someone in your life to practise with, in imagination. It could be a friend, family member, client, stranger or work colleague.

◇ Imagine that you are in the presence of that person, practising being totally *non-judging* of them – for one day, one week, one month, one year.

Exercise 3:

Living Mindfully by Non-striving

How can I do this exercise?

◇ Return to Chapter 11 and read through again the description given there for living with an attitude of *Non-striving*.

◇ Find a quiet time and place.

◇ Spend a few minutes reading through the poem below, reflecting on each line, imagining as best you can what it would be like to live each moment with an attitude of *non-striving* in all of the images that come into your mind – giving 100 percent, but not straining; not competing, just aiming for the very best.

> The sun gives us exactly the right heat –
> striving to do more would surely end us all.
> The flute being played
> does not try to change the tune –
> it seeks only to be straight and hollow
> so the best sound can always be heard.
>
> There is a dance to be danced through us –
> we don't have to try to dance.
> There is a measured beat
> to which we can march –
> not one that can be heard
> but one that says, "Let go of striving.
> Just follow the prompting of the heart."

◇ Think of someone in your life to practise with, in imagination. It could be a friend, family member, client, stranger or work colleague.

◇ Imagine that you are in the presence of that person, practising being totally *non-striving* in your interaction with them – for one day, one week, one month, one year.

<u>Exercise 4:</u>
Living Mindfully with Trust

How can I do this exercise?

◇ Return to Chapter 11 and read through again the description given there for living with an attitude of *Trust.*

◇ Find a quiet time and place.

◇ Spend a few minutes reading through the poem below, reflecting on each line, imagining as best you can what it would be like to live each moment with full *trust* in all of the images that come into your mind.

> One who lives in trust
> does not doubt the perfection of things,
> that all is proceeding according to a Higher Plan,
> and that everything is either good
> or leading towards the good.

◇ Think of someone in your life to practise with, in imagination. It could be a friend, family member, client, stranger or work colleague.

◇ Imagine that you are in the presence of that person, practising having full *trust* in your interaction with them – for one day, one week, one month, one year.

Exercise 5:

Living Mindfully by Letting Go

How can I do this exercise ?

◇ Return to Chapter 11 and read through again the description given there for living with an attitude of *Letting go.*

◇ Find a quiet time and place.

◇ Spend a few minutes reading through the poem below, reflecting on each line, imagining as best you can what it would be like to live with total *letting go* in all of the images that come into your mind.

> If we can let go of the past,
> it is seen as but a dream.
>
> If we can let go of the future,
> the delight of the present is always here.
>
> If we can let go of wanting,
> we find the treasure within.
>
> Forgetting the help we have given to others,
> and forgetting the harm others have done to us.

If we can let go of thinking,
our mind will be free.

◇ Think of someone in your life to practise with, in imagination. It could be a friend, family member, client, stranger or work colleague.

◇ Imagine that you are in the presence of that person, practising *letting go* in your interaction with them – for one day, one week, one month, one year.

Exercise 6:
Living Mindfully with a Beginner's Mind

How can I do this exercise?

◇ Return to Chapter 11 and read through again the description given there for living with an attitude of *Beginner's Mind*.

◇ Find a quiet time and place.

◇ Spend a few minutes reading the poem below, reflecting on each line, imagining as best you can what it would be like to live with a *beginner's mind* in all of the images that come into your mind.

Everything is seen for the very first time;
every sound is totally new;
all movement was not there before;
every sensation is always the first.

Let us feel that we are born
with the dawn of each new day.

◇ Think of someone in your life to practise with, in imagination. It could be a friend, family member, client, stranger or work colleague.

◇ Imagine that you are in the presence of that person, practising having a *beginner's mind* in your interaction with them – for one day, one week, one month, one year.

<u>Exercise 7:</u>
Living Mindfully with Patience

How can I do this exercise?

◇ Return to Chapter 11 and read through again the description given there for living with an attitude of *Patience*.

◇ Find a quiet time and place.

◇ Spend a few minutes reading the poem below, reflecting on each line, imagining as best you can what it would be like to live every moment with complete *patience* in all of the images that come into your mind.

> The sun rises up at exactly the right time,
> and so too the tide goes not out early.
> Some flowers on the bush come easily first
> while others are the very long last -
> the timing of each one is perfection.
>
> It takes courage to be patient
> yet it's impatience that makes us brave.
> Let us live in patience,
> knowing that everything is happening,
> and will happen, at exactly the right time.

◇ Think of someone in your life to practise with, in imagination. It could be a friend, family member, client, stranger or work colleague.

◇ Imagine that you are in the presence of that person, practising *patience* in your interaction with them – for one day, one week, one month, one year.

Exercise 8:

The Prayer of Compassion

When we repeat a prayer a few times in a quiet, gentle, reflective manner, our mind becomes still and our heart begins to open in joy, love and compassion. An awareness grows of our Peaceful Mind, Open Heart. We begin to live in the timeless moment of intoning the prayer, becoming absorbed in the opening of the heart.

This prayer is suitable for every circumstance – for people who are dying as well as for those who are healthy; for those who are young as well as for the old; for people in pain and suffering and those who feel quite content. It can be a useful exercise for us as we age. Whatever our circumstance, whatever our age or state of health, we can wish happiness for ourselves and for others.

How can I do this exercise?

◇ This is the version of the Prayer of Compassion recommended for aging gracefully:
  - As I grow older, may I be kind to myself.
  - As I grow older, may I accept joy and sorrow.
  - As I grow older, may I be happy and at peace.

As you say it a few times to yourself, feel how the opening of your heart is generating compassion.

◇ Now share the compassion with others. Think of people you are close to, or work with, or are connected with. Think of them and say the prayer in this way a few times:

- As each of us grows older, may we be kind to ourselves.
- As each of us grows older, may we accept joy and sorrow.
- As each of us grows older, may we be happy and at peace.

◇ Now we share this wish with all those in the world who are with us on the aging journey. It is never a journey that we take alone. Everyone we know is aging; everyone in the world is aging. Think of all people everywhere and say the prayer in this way a few times:

- As all beings grow older, may they be kind to themselves.
- As all beings grow older, may they accept joy and sorrow.
- As all beings grow older, may they be happy and at peace.

And I have felt ...
a sense sublime of something far more deeply interfused
Whose dwelling is the light of setting suns,
And the round ocean and the living air,
And the blue sky, and in the mind of man;
A motion and a spirit, that impels
All thinking things, all objects of all thought,
And rolls through all things.

William Wordsworth

Part Five

Becoming a Compassionate Carer Along the Path of Aging

Don't think
the garden
loses its
ecstasy in
winter.
It's quiet,
but the
roots are
down there
riotous.

Jalaluddin Rumi

Chapter 13

Becoming a Compassionate Carer

Caring about others, running the risk of feeling,
and leaving an impact on people,
brings happiness.

Rabbi Harold Kushner

Apart from the devastation wrought by the Spanish Flu pandemic and the two World Wars, there was a steady increase in life expectancy during the last century, with a corresponding reduction in new births as the standard of living rose in industrialised countries. Although the age of dying moved into the 80's and 90's, this longer life span did not guarantee a healthy old age. The number of people who live in residential aged care facilities has increased and this trend is expected to accelerate over time. Residents of aged care facilities are also characterised as having more complex health needs, a pattern which is also predicted to continue to increase. As such, providing good care for the expanding aging population has been a challenge for healthcare systems worldwide.

When older people are able to remain living in their own home or with family members, the vast majority of care is provided by the spouse or adult children. As the older share of population increases and people live longer with chronic disabling conditions, meeting the care needs will become more challenging.

While most of the research indicates that opening our heart in compassion and putting the needs of the suffering before our own has a beneficial effect upon the carer, prolonged caregiving appears to take a toll on their physical and mental health. We will explore the reasons for this as we go along.

Role of a Compassionate Caregiver

As we journey through life, many of us already are, or will become, a caregiver in some form or another. Perhaps we are caring for our aging partner or child with special needs, looking after one or both of our elderly parents, or giving up our time and energy to help others in need. And some will be working as community nurses or professionals in residential aged care facilities, hospices and other places of care.

A caregiver is anyone who takes care of those who are not able to look after themselves, whether it be due to a medical condition (physical disabilities, strokes, accidents) or to mental health deterioration such as depression or dementia. The term applies equally to professionals, family members, friends and volunteers, regardless of where the caring takes place.

Apart from the very real demands for physical and medical care, as compassionate caregivers we are committed to doing all that we can to assist the one in need to reconnect with their Peaceful Mind, Open Heart – that is, to rediscover those deeper layers of our innate Human Values of Love, Truth, Peace, Right Conduct and Non-violence ever-waiting within. How is this to be done? The path that we are recommending is best illustrated by the acronym CARER:

C	Compassionate Heart
A	Awareness of Oneness
R	Regulation of Self
E	Environment
R	Resilience

Let us explore in turn each one of these five defining characteristics of the compassionate carer.

Compassionate Heart

Until the advent of modern medicine the compassionate heart had always been considered throughout history to be the key to quality caring. For whatever reason, the rapid advances in medical science and training brought with it a form of professional detachment that often precluded tenderness, loving care and compassion. However, this attitude is now changing because of the recent developments in neuroscience and positive psychology demonstrating the powerful healing qualities of compassion, gratitude, positivity and loving-kindness.

Neuroscientist Mary Helen Immordino-Yang and her colleagues proposed in their 2009 research paper, *Neural Correlates of Admiration and Compassion*, that someone who cares in a compassionate way is linking at a neuronal level their interoceptive sensations, emotions, exteroceptive connections and rational thought. That is, when we are behaving in a compassionate way, the emotional and rational parts of our brain are inextricably linked.

While empathy is the capacity to sense the inner state of another person, compassion is the wish that they not suffer and includes the urge to do something to bring relief. Some researchers in the field have proposed that our inborn wish to connect with others is what facilitates the feeling of empathy. Through experiencing the pathos of their condition, there arises within us a sense of identification with the person, and this provides the motivation to do something to relieve their suffering, out of compassion.

In a literal sense, compassion means to 'suffer with'. It is thought that, for compassion to reach its full strength as a motivating force to help others, we would have to be able to feel what the other is going through to the fullest extent possible. This means that we need to be able to make room for another's feelings within ourselves, and to be comfortable with that discomfort, regarding it with the same detachment as the cinema screen being aware of the fleeting images of suffering projected onto its surface while the movie drama unfolds. If we are not able to regard our feelings in this dispassionate way, when those waves of compassion roll in on us one after the other, there can be a growing anxiety, a creeping depression or a flattening of affect, indicating that we are not able to cope with any more suffering . The question is, how do we as the compassionate carer deal with and regulate such intensity of emotion without detriment to ourselves?

For those engaged in helping others in places where the suffering is on-going and relentless, neuropsychiatrists and positive psychologists advise that it is through the expression of Love-filled virtues that the empathic burden can be relieved. That is, by engaging in a thousand little acts of kindness, love, generosity, respect, patience and understanding, the fire in our heart is put to good use instead of burning the forest down inside. These qualities define the Human Value of Love, the unconditional love that is as endless in its outpouring as the rays from the sun. It is an adventure of the heart, a willingness to let ourselves be transformed into a conduit for Love, an instrument to be played by the Higher Good that guides the whole universe. And, as we change, those in our care will feel the warmth of our Sun, bringing relief to the cold winter that may have been blanketing their hearts.

Cultivating compassion in our life and in our role as a care provider

The obvious benefit to us of increasing the level of compassion in our lives – both for others and for ourselves – is that it helps us to be happier, opening our heart and giving us a sense of meaning and purpose, and it promotes happiness in those around us as well. However, some research studies indicate that bringing more compassion into our lives also brings other unexpected rewards. For example, people who practise developing compassion produce 100 percent more DHEA, which is a hormone that counteracts the aging process, and 23 percent less cortisol, known as the 'stress hormone'.

Knowing that each one of us, without exception, wants to be more happy, less stressed and to age gently, gives us an additional incentive to cultivate and practise compassion every day in our home lives and in our role as a carer.

Further, remembering that the Human Value of Love is the essential ingredient for all of the other noble virtues, it follows from esoteric spiritual teachings that each time we open our heart in compassion we come closer to living in the realms of our higher Self. Matt Valentine, in his 2016 book, *Living Zen Spirit,* recommended that:

> *By working to express compassion towards others, we realize the true nature of our existence and discover a deep sense of peace and happiness.*

University of Wisconsin neuropsychiatrist Richard Davidson's research on Tibetan Buddhist monks in 2008 found that meditating on compassion can produce powerful changes in the brain. In his research paper, *Buddha's Brain: Neuroplasticity and Meditation*, Davidson said that, when the monks were asked to meditate on unconditional loving-kindness and compassion, their brains generated powerful gamma waves that may have indicated a compassionate state of mind. The study provides evidence that we might be able to increase empathy by exercising the brain with a loving-kindness meditation.

A 2013 study from Harvard and Northeastern University, conducted by psychologists David DeSteno and Paul Condon, supported this finding, demonstrating that participants who had meditated were more likely than non-meditators to lend a helping hand to an actor with crutches who was pretending to be in pain.

Whether it be through special meditations, or sheer courage to feel the joys and sorrows of others, we know that the neural networks in our brain that support compassion can be increased through our taking repeated steps in this direction. At first it might seem that we are doing this for the sake of the sufferers, but really we are doing it for ourselves, to come closer to experiencing who we truly are – an ever-blissful, purely loving, ever-content human being.

Awareness of Oneness

The Human Values of Love and Truth are, at their highest level, manifestations of Oneness, of the underlying unity of all seemingly separate things. This is where spirituality coalesces with the science of quantum physics, as we will see.

According to the Human Values philosophy offered in this Handbook, we will not be able to love others in the most pure way as long as we regard them as different from each other, and from ourselves. This might well sound strange at first and requires analogies and metaphors to illustrate its meaning.

Consider this: The eyelid would not be motivated to protect the eye – particularly when at risk of damage to itself from the intruding finger or projectile – if it regarded itself as separate from the eye. It protects the eye because both eyelid and eye are part of the one body. Similarly the tongue does not seek revenge against the clumsy teeth that have bitten into it; and the bruised hand will not punish the other hand for wielding the hammer that hit the thumb instead of the roofing nail. And why not? Of course the answer is clear: because the tongue and the teeth, and both of the hands, belong to the one body.

Other metaphors are manifold. For example, the eye warns the feet when a thorn lies on the pathway; the stomach works hard to process food, for the sake of the whole body; and the tiny heart organ beats over 100,000 times a day, pumping blood through the circulatory system over a journey of 32,000 kilometres in any 24 hour period, not for itself but purely for the sake of the estimated 100 billion neurons in the brain and the 100,000 billion cells in the body. Each part of the body is constantly engaged in loving, selfless service to the rest of the body. The human body itself demonstrates that Love is present at the highest level when there is an awareness of Oneness.

This Oneness describes, in part, the Human Value of Truth. That is, the differences between us only seem to be real, in the same way that waves on the one vast ocean only appear to be separate from each other – they are merely transient changes in the form of the one sea. As well as the metaphor of the ocean there are many others we can use to illustrate our essential Oneness:

- There are many different shapes and colours of light bulbs, but the one electricity illuminates them all.
- The one lump of clay can be moulded into creating many different cups, plates and bowls, but the clay in all of them is the same. Broken down, all form into the one lump of clay.
- Similarly, a bar of gold can be shaped into various ornaments, some (the Royal crown) seemingly more important than others (the anklet), but the gold in all is the same. Melted down, they reveal their essential oneness yet again.

The feeling of Oneness is not something that can be arrived at overnight. There is a saying: 'First the mind, then the heart will follow'. We will have to train our mind to think in this all-is-one way. Living in this age of science allows us to put aside much of our scepticism because renowned theoretical physicists in the past 100 years have been assuring us that there is essentially no difference between one object and another, that all are waves on an unimaginably vast ocean of energy. Albert Einstein wrote:

A human being is part of the whole, called by us, 'Universe', a part limited in time and space. He experiences himself, his thoughts and feelings as something separated from the rest – a kind of optical delusion of his consciousness. This delusion is a kind of prison for us, restricting us to our personal desires and to affection for a few persons nearest to us. Our task must be to free ourselves from this prison by widening our circle of compassion to embrace all living creatures and the whole of nature in its beauty.

With the help of metaphors and the permission to be open-minded given by quantum physics, we can accept that we are in fact all one, only apparently separate from each other. It is a paradox – which the right side of our brain is comfortable with – in that we are both separate and not separate. The more we are mindful of thinking that we are all one, the easier it is for the heart to open fully in love for another. Then, the more we love, the more it becomes real that we are in fact all one. As Sathya Sai Baba said:

Seen through the eyes of Love,
all beings are beautiful,
all deeds are dedicated,
all thoughts are innocent.
The world is one vast kin.

As compassionate carers we already do our best to love and enrich the lives of each and every person under our care to the same degree. However it is not always easy to do this. Most of us would find our heart freezing up when a foul-mouthed, abusive, unhappy person ridicules our sincere efforts to be a good carer. So how are we to achieve this high aim?

To our minds the first step is to believe (or at least be open to believing) that within each one of us is a 'diamond' covered by varying degrees of 'mud'. The aim is to look for this diamond both within ourselves and in each person we interact with. We can remind ourselves that divinity – the five

Human Values, the Spirit – lies equally within all those in our care, as does the one current of electricity illuminate each of the many different light bulbs.

Having convinced ourselves of the veracity of thinking in this way, compassion can then flow towards the person who is mentally impaired, abusive or disruptive. We can remember that unfortunate circumstances can conspire to cover our diamond – our Peaceful Mind, Open Heart – with the mud of mental deterioration, indifference, self-doubt and abuse.

If, on the other hand, we allow ourselves to think, "This person is angry. I'll not waste time on him," we will be denying him the opportunity to change, to align himself with the Human Values that are his birthright. We will be denying him the possibility of a radical transformation, because we ourselves have not changed. As long as we see only the outer differences, the transforming power of our Love cannot touch him.

Let us believe that each person's Essence is calling to us to bring It forth, to make it manifest. Let us believe that all are One, that all are divine. Then we can care with true compassion.

Regulation of Self

To become a compassionate caregiver, we will need to learn how to regulate our habitual (often unconscious) patterns of thinking, sensing, feeling and action – that is, to become the master instead of the slave of this vehicle that we move around in, so that we can live according to our innate Human Values. Self-regulation is only possible if first we have self-awareness. If we have current information about how this human robot is already programmed, we are then in a position to change the program, to self-regulate, to change the course of the river of our life.

In the earlier part of this book we saw that self-regulation can be engaged in by focussing on one or more of the three pathways of Reflection, Resilience and Relationship.

To be an effective compassionate carer, we need to be able to find our Centre (our Peaceful Mind, Open Heart; our higher Self), to nurture our Centre and keep the balance in our connections with ourself and with others. There needs to be harmony between our thoughts, words and deeds. Unless these three are in concert with each other, and accord with the five Human Values, all attempts at being an effective compassionate carer will be weakened. Sathya Sai Baba has advised:

> *All thoughts arise from the heart and lead to actions. Hence for all thoughts, words and deeds, the heart is the source. What should be the condition of the heart? It should be full of compassion.*

Although there are as yet no neuropsychological research studies to support this assertion, it is in accord with the words and writings of several wise souls such as the 14th Dalai Lama, Jalaluddin Rumi, Sri Aurobindo, Ralph Waldo Emerson and others. As a result we can say that the first challenge for us in becoming compassionate carers is to ensure that every thought arising into consciousness is vetted as to its alignment with the five Human Values. Is it loving, kind, compassionate, selfless or grateful? Will it enhance peace, equanimity, patience and forbearance? Does this thought promote open-mindedness, humility, integrity and self-honesty? Is it in accord with my conscience, and is there any trace of anger, annoyance, judgment or resentment in this thought?

If the thought is not pure in that sense, it is to be let go of – or even forcibly expelled if necessary. When common sense and loving thoughts arise they can be held on to, contemplated on, spoken or otherwise acted upon.

With such diligent mindfulness we can prepare the ground for the seeds of empathy, compassion and loving-kindness to sprout and grow strong.

Environment

We know from a number of research studies that our environment contributes enormously to our health, happiness, and ability to learn. Our own experience tells us that when we have healthy nutrition, moderate exercise, good sleep, and when our living space is clean, tidy, bright and close to Nature in some way, we function better and our mood is lighter.

Being a compassionate carer means being able to imagine ourselves in the shoes of the one we are looking after, asking, "What environment would I like to live in so that I can find happiness and a sense of purpose in being alive?" Researchers, psychologists, nurses and doctors, such as Atul Gawande who wrote *Being Mortal,* have listed a number of essential attributes of an environment that will nurture and promote life satisfaction and wellbeing in those who need care. The ideal environment is one that:

- Diminishes fears and anxiety about suffering and death
- Increases coping skills
- Restores or maintains dignity and a sense of personhood
- Maintains and develops interpersonal, reciprocal heart-to-heart connections
- Allows one to find a sense of meaning, purpose and acceptance in life

As will be explained later in this chapter, another important attribute of an environment that has a rejuvenating effect upon those in care is where the elements of Nature are brought into the home. A fine example of this is SWAMI Home in Singapore which has leafy gardens, running-water ponds stocked with coloured fish, areas open to the sunshine, and the complete absence of any offensive odours. Other compassionate environments include indoor growing plants, dogs, cats, birds, and frequent visits by children from local schools.

Researchers have discovered the rejuvenating and healing power of: posters with values-based words such as 'Love all. Serve all' and 'Seeing you brings joy to my heart'; playing certain classical music pieces such as those by Bach and Mozart; spiritual chanting and heart-opening instrumental music.

Resilience

As was discussed earlier, the compassionate carer will need to develop a high level of resilience. Without this, there is the possibility of *compassion fatigue*, characterised by a gradual lessening of compassion over time. Sufferers of compassion fatigue can have feelings of hopelessness, a decrease in experiences of pleasure, sleeplessness, chronic stress and anxiety. It has been called the *cost of caring*, the cost that we pay for caring for those whose suffering is continuous and unresolvable.

What is thought to happen is that, when we are being confronted with abject suffering in others on a daily basis, our inclination to be empathic and helpful can work against us if we do not have sufficient resilience to deal with such pathos.

You will recall that we explored the topic of resilience in Chapter 3 in some detail. The approaches given there (the Five C's of Resilient Coping, the BOUNCE BACK program, and the Healthy Mind Platter) are well-supported by a number of research studies. In addition to that material, let's look more closely at how compassionate caregivers can safely allow themselves to remain empathic and motivated to relieve the suffering of others with joy and an open heart.

Our concern here is one of how to avoid becoming overwhelmed by feelings of powerlessness, helplessness and despair, and being overcome by the immensity of the task, perhaps drifting into depression and indifference.

It helps to reflect on the lives of historical figures who have demonstrated the ability to not only cope with but to thrive in the midst of the most appalling suffering. Our such person was Mother Teresa whose committed task was to assist those dying alone on the streets of Calcutta, arranging for them to be loved and comforted during their final hours in a hospice. When asked how she managed to cope, she replied, "When I see a poverty-stricken person dying of the most terrible disease, I see Jesus with a cold." In other words, within each suffering person, Mother Teresa saw or believed there to be a divine Being, one who regarded the body's suffering as no more than having a cold. There is a saying:

> When I am identified
> With my higher Self,
> With the deathless Self that I am,
> I am ever-content,
> For grief and anxiety
> Can never affect me,
> And fear can never enter me.

When we remember that the eternal Spirit residing in each suffering person is not affected by their ordeal, we can do our best to minimize their distress, while at the same time knowing that the screen is not affected by the movie.

Further, we know from our own trials and travails that all suffering gives an opportunity for awakening to deeper levels of Peaceful Mind, Open Heart within ourselves. The Lebanese poet Kahlil Gibran wrote, "Your pain is the breaking of the shell that encloses your understanding." The philosophy underlying the Human Values approach recommends that the compassionate carer holds on to the conviction that, whatever the terror and suffering endured by the ones we are caring for, in due course they will find a way of transmuting their base metal into gold, of tasting their own sweet sugar arising from the burning and crushing of the sugarcane.

Of course we can only believe in this for others if we are already well-practised in regarding our own struggles and agonies as just more grist for the mill, the crushing of the grain to give us the riches of fine flour.

One further resilience attitude recommended for the compassionate carer is to let go of the belief that we have any real power to reduce the suffering of others, yet at the same time behaving as if we have absolute power to do so. There is safety in such paradoxes – they allow us to be empathic to the full and to love unreservedly, without being exhausted by the assumption that we are the ones playing this flute, doing this dance, tending to this flower.

Approaches in Caring for the Aged in Residential Settings

Person-centered approach to care

Carl Rogers, one of the 20th century's most influential humanistic psychologists, proposed that a *person-centered* approach, based on acceptance, caring, empathy, sensitivity, and active listening, promotes optimal personal growth. He believed that, in order to maximize their potential in late life, individuals should have access to, and opportunities for, ongoing learning, personal challenges, and close and intimate relationships. Furthermore, he argued that the human capacity for growth does not diminish with age, nor does the need for growth become less relevant as we age. The emphasis in person-centered care is on the well-being and quality of life as defined by the individual we are caring for.

In 1991, William Thomas, a US geriatrician, pioneered the *Eden Alternative*, which is a person-centered approach to long-term residential aged care. His central premise was that: "Every creature has a habitat in which it thrives, and one in which it withers. Human beings wither in institutions."

Like Rogers, Thomas believed that late life was an active phase of the aging trajectory, and to that end he wanted to create a human habitat that would optimise growth for long-term care residents. His aim was to deinstitutionalize aged care facilities by enlivening the environment with children, animals, and plants to create an atmosphere reminiscent of home. The Eden Alternative is based on a set of principles to create a warm and caring environment that enriches the lives of all who live and work in it.

In her 2012 book, *The Heart of Care – Dignity in Action: A Guide to Person-Centred Compassionate Elder Care*, Amanda Waring emphasized that caring for our elders is sacred work that should have preserving the essence of human dignity at its heart. She recommended the following nine roles for us to play:

1. We will need to cultivate an ability to listen, appreciate, empathise and celebrate.
2. We will need to look at the world from the perspective of an older person.
3. We will need to recognise, address and pacify our own fears.
4. We will need to examine our own attitudes to and assumptions about older people.
5. We will need to develop compassion and deep awareness of the suffering of another, coupled with the desire to relieve it.
6. We will need to practise self-care, self-love, self-responsibility and self-knowledge.
7. We will need to keep motivated, to sustain morale and not lose our sense of humour.
8. We will need to be brave enough and honest enough to ask for help.
9. We will need to look at how we can respect wishes, offer choices and give back a sense of control where appropriate.

Peaceful Mind, Open Heart in aged care facilities

For many of the elderly, particularly those who require full-time nursing care, it is as if the light and warmth has gone out of their lives. They are like the fallen branches of humanity's tree, waiting or even hoping for their final transition.

In taking up our role as a compassionate carer, we can become like blazing logs, afire with the five Human Values, radiating Peaceful Mind and Open Heart. To the extent that we can master this art of self-transformation, those in our care will also find a light within themselves, one that burns gently and kindly with a new joy and purpose in remaining alive inside a body that is breaking down, decaying with age.

To give carers a guide on how to be mindful in integrating the philosophy of Peaceful Mind and Open Heart into their work, we have developed a Carer's Code of Conduct based on the five universal Human Values. The Code advises that, as a convenient checklist:

Love can be expressed by:

- ◇ Relating to the 'wise inner-goodness' of each person in our care
- ◇ Whenever possible, putting the interests of the person ahead of our own
- ◇ Using caring and respectful words
- ◇ Developing compassion, so that the other's pain and frustration is felt and understood

Peace can be expressed by:

- ◇ Being a good listener
- ◇ Taking time to explain things carefully, sometimes more than once
- ◇ Showing patience and tolerance, even when provoked
- ◇ Moving without hurry or haste

Truth can be expressed by:

- ◇ Practising honesty in dealing with staff and the people we are caring for
- ◇ Recognising that we are more than a body that moves, thinks and feels – that we are all kings and queens in disguise
- ◇ Learning to discover and trust our own intuition
- ◇ Developing self-confidence and having trust in a higher power

Right Conduct can be expressed by:

- ◇ Behaving towards others (particularly those we are caring for) as one would like others to behave towards us
- ◇ Demonstrating personal tidiness, punctuality and integrity
- ◇ Being true to the dictates of our own conscience
- ◇ Having respect for society's laws, the elderly, our parents, and for the customs and practices of other cultures and faiths

Non-violence can be expressed by:

- ◇ Refraining from using hurtful words or actions
- ◇ Not speaking (or thinking) badly about others
- ◇ Speaking gently and kindly, even when firmness is required
- ◇ Avoiding the expression of our own anger, resentment, bitterness, jealousy and selfishness – changing them into love and peace as much as we can

Only the development of
compassion and understanding for others
can bring us the tranquillity and happiness we seek.

14th Dalai Lama

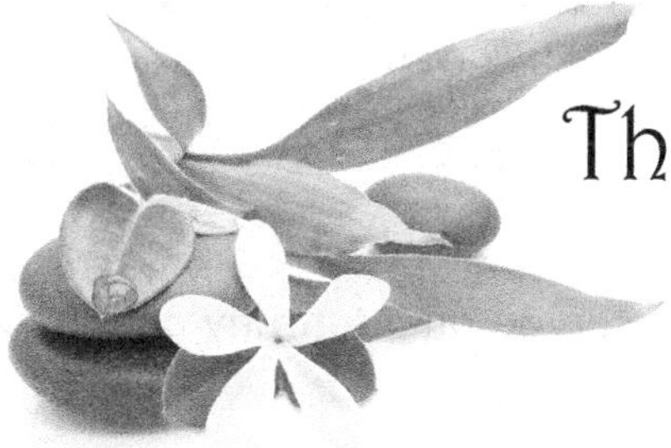

The Practice

EXERCISES FOR CULTIVATING COMPASSION

All of us to varying degrees have experienced deep compassion for someone who was suffering, doing whatever we can to be of some help. Yet, at other times, we can hear of some calamity or see people suffering on the television news channel and the feeling of compassion is just fleeting, soon replaced by other thoughts, or perhaps there was not even a hint of empathy triggered by what we've just heard or seen. If we want to have compassion arise in us with the same fullness as a loving mother responding to the cries of her child, it will take practice using different forms of meditation, guided imagination and mindfulness.

We were born with compassion. It is just that life's circumstances have transpired to cover it up, like ash covering a fire. When we practise methods like the loving-kindness meditation, this removes the ash from the fire, little by little, until there is a forest fire of compassion inside us, waiting to spread its light and warmth to all sentient beings who might be suffering.

Exercise 1:
Developing Compassion Through CARER

This is a guided imagination that you can do with eyes open or closed, whichever is comfortable. We will be using the imagination to grow those neuronal circuits in the brain that support compassion, with a focus on each component of the acronym CARER (Compassionate Heart, Awareness of Oneness, Regulation of Self, Environment, Resilience).

How can I do this exercise?

◇ Find a quiet time and place when you can go on a journey of imagination.

◇ Imagine what it would be like if you had gone through many years of practice, and now your *heart was full of compassion*.

◇ Imagine that you could feel all of the pain and suffering of just one person you know, but without being upset by it. It's like you are the movie screen and the suffering is being projected onto your surface.

◇ Now imagine sending streams of love to this person, wishing that your love will erase all of their suffering.

◇ Imagine also that you are giving loving, practical help to them, all with a prayer that this will help them to be free of suffering.

◇ Now imagine doing this for two or more people – feeling their pain and sending healing love and a prayer. This love comes from an inexhaustible supply within you.

◇ Imagine doing this for more and more people, sending your love and your prayers to heal their suffering. Feel your heart expanding with compassion.

◇ Now we'll imagine what it would be like to have an *awareness of oneness*.

◇ Imagine what it would be like to feel a sense of unity or oneness with everybody and everything. To do this, imagine that each person that you know is like a wave on the one vast ocean. All waves are part of the same ocean. Imagine using that image to feel Oneness with everyone and everything.

◇ Imagine what it would be like if you had been practising the 'wave and the sea' imagination for one week, for a month, for a whole year. Imagine what it would be like feeling that Oneness with everybody and everything, particularly in your role as a carer.

◇ Imagine that you have been applying all that you can understand about *regulation* of your thoughts, feelings and actions. Imagine that you are now master of your mind, body and feelings. Imagine yourself being able to regulate all aspects of your personality so as to be able to live the Human Values of Love, Truth, Peace, Right Conduct and Non-violence at a very advanced level, particularly in your role as a carer.

◇ Now imagine the *environment* that you would like to create, both in your home and work situation.

◇ Imagine that you have created the ideal environment, particularly in roles where you are caring for others. Let your imagination have total freedom to be creative.

◇ Now we'll imagine what it would be like to have the upmost *resilience*.

◇ Imagine that you've been studying and practising the Five C's of Resilient Coping, the BOUNCE BACK program and the Healthy Mind Platter, for one year. Imagine how resilient you would be. Imagine being totally at ease in any situation, totally resilient, particularly in your role as a carer.

◇ Now imagine that you are living your life as a compassionate carer, being exemplary in the five areas of:

Compassionate Heart
Awareness of Oneness
Regulation of Self
Environment
Resilience

<u>Exercise 2:</u>
Living the Carer's Code of Conduct

How can I do this exercise?

- ◇ Read again the Carer's Code of Conduct in this chapter (pages 249, 250).
- ◇ Reflecting back over the past week, give yourself a rating of 1 to 5 for each one of the four conduct guidelines for each of the five Human Values, where 1 represents 'Not at all' and 5 represents 'Doing exceptionally well'.
- ◇ Identify the lowest-rated guideline (choose one if there are two or more lowest), over all of the Human Values.
- ◇ Create an action plan for improving the quality of your compassionate caring, for that particular conduct guideline, and apply it for one to two weeks.
- ◇ When you are satisfied with your progress for that guideline, identify the next lowest, and create an action plan.
- ◇ You can continue to do this for as long as you wish, using the Code of Conduct questionnaire as a convenient checklist for self analysis.
- ◇ After 3 to 6 months, you might like to complete the Code of Conduct checklist again, to look at your progress in self-transformation, the extent to which you live the Human Values in your caregiver role.

Exercise 3:
Windows of the Soul

This is an exercise to give practice in allowing more of our innate compassion to rise up within us. It is carried out with a partner.

How I can do this exercise?

- ◇ Find a partner to practise with who is willing to explore how to connect with deeper levels of compassion. You can read each step of the instructions aloud, for both of you.
- ◇ Sit opposite each other, and look into the eyes of your partner.
- ◇ Allow the feeling of compassion to shine through your eyes.
- ◇ You are not having to fix anything, say anything or do anything – just maintain a soft gaze with your partner.
- ◇ If you feel embarrassed, let that feeling pass – just breathe and be with the other person, holding eye contact.
- ◇ Check how you are feeling. Do you feel a deeper connection with the person opposite you? Can you feel their emotion and their needs?
- ◇ After five minutes of practice, discuss with each other what you experienced.
- ◇ The next time you are with an elder or someone else in your care, allow some eye contact and see if you can repeat what you have practised here. You'll be actively relaxed and fully present, remembering that you don't need to provide solutions or answers – just allowing yourself to be fully present with the person is enough, allowing compassion to shine through your eyes.

Exercise 4:

Empathy and Compassion for Those in Care

This is an exercise using our imagination. It can be a very moving experience and worthwhile repeating every week or so for a while. You can record the instructions and listen to them alone, or you can ask someone to read them to you, using appropriate pauses to allow deeper levels of empathy and compassion to be experienced.

How can I do this exercise?

- ◇ Find a quiet time and place for the next 5 to 10 minutes.
- ◇ Using a self-created recording, or having a friend read them to you, these are the instructions for the guided imagination.
- ◇ Close your eyes and imagine. Imagine that you have experienced some trauma that has left you unable to move any part of your body except your hand.
- ◇ Imagine that you are now living in a nursing home, and you are dependent upon the care of others for all of your basic needs.
- ◇ Imagine that the carers have given you your breakfast, cleaned you up, dressed you and put you in a wheelchair. They have wheeled you out of your room and left you in front of the nurse's station.
- ◇ Imagine that all you can see is the top of the nurse's head as she leans down to write. Occasionally you can see people scurrying by as they go about their duties – what you see is mostly their feet and knees.
- ◇ Imagine that you can hear the phone ringing and the nurse answering it. You can hear the staff chattering and laughing, the intercom blaring out a message, and the sound of a noisy floor polisher.
- ◇ Now imagine that you have been sitting here for an hour ... now two hours ... You are so tired that you are no longer able to hold up your head.
- ◇ Imagine if this was your life for two months ... for two years ... for longer.

◇ Now that you can feel what it might be like for such a person, allow sweet, loving compassion for them to rise up in your heart.
◇ Imagine hundreds of rays of your compassion beaming out of you and touching someone just like you imagined. Imagine your compassion filling every atom and cell in their body, so that they feel truly loved.

<u>Exercise 5:</u>
Nurturing Compassion for all Beings

The more we can practise nurturing and growing compassion, with more and more people, animals and living things, the more will we find ourselves radiating compassion whenever we are with or even hear about others who are suffering in some way.

How can I do this exercise?

◇ Find a quiet time and place, to imagine.
◇ Begin with a focus on your breath. Breathe calmly and naturally, and concentrate all of your attention on the movements of the breath.
◇ Keep returning your attention to the breath. If thoughts come, just let them go, and return your attention to the breath.
◇ Now we will begin opening the doors to your compassionate heart.
◇ Imagine that someone close to you has had a serious accident, and is now suffering terrible pain. Imagine that you have such a strong empathic connection to this person that you can feel all of the pain they are going through, all of their fear and suffering.
◇ Now imagine that a limitless feeling of love for this person is rising up in you. Imagine that streams of this pure sweet love are flowing out of you and going into this cherished person.
◇ Visualise that every atom of this person's suffering is now replaced by an atom of love. Every atom and cell in them is now filled with love.
◇ Wish from the bottom of your heart that your friend survives, gets

better, and suffers no more.

- ◇ Now extend this warm, loving compassion to other beings who are close to you; then, little by little, extend this compassion to all beings, imagining all of them being surrounded by and filled with your loving compassion.
- ◇ Now create this wish from the bottom of your heart and beam it out far and wide:

May all beings be freed from suffering and
from the causes of their suffering.

- ◇ Silently repeat this wish a few times.

To laugh often and much;
To win the respect of intelligent people
and the affection of children ...
To appreciate beauty;
To find the best in others;
To leave the world a bit better,
whether by a healthy child,
a garden patch, or a redeemed social condition;
To know that even one life
has breathed easier because you have lived.
This is to have succeeded.

Ralph Waldo Emerson

Chapter 14

Managing the Challenges of Caring for the Aged

It is not how much you do, but how much
Love you put in the doing.

Mother Teresa

To a large extent, those entering the Fourth Age (85+ years) do not yet stand out as an issue that society has to come to terms with. Seldom venturing out because it is easier to stay at home, they remain largely unseen. However the sobering reality is presented to us by the reports of several national Bureaus of Statistics, indicating that aging brings with it an increased likelihood of disability and the need for assistance with the basic activities of daily living. These facts are beginning to play their part in raising society's awareness of families in crisis in caring for the aged, a crisis that will not only affect the health and wellbeing of family members and professional caregivers, but also the health care services as a whole. Clearly, we are not ready for such a tidal wave of increased responsibility at this time.

The challenge is further compounded when we look into how the incidence of mental illness is rising steadily amongst the aged. Common mental disorders such as depression, anxiety and dementia make it difficult for the elderly person to maintain their personal care, engage in housework and organise finances and social activity. Those caring for the aged who have mental and emotional problems are faced with obstacles and hardships far beyond those arising when physical disability alone is present.

Unless we have experienced it ourselves, we cannot fully grasp how difficult it must be for loved ones, in particular, to be not only grieving for what their beloved is struggling with, but also having to face their own fears of how they would cope with being disabled, dependent, ill and dying. Couple all of that with sheer physical exhaustion, and we have a mountain that is very steep to climb and easy to fall down from.

Depression and Anxiety

Although many people think that depression is a normal part of aging, according to research findings given in the 2008 *Oxford Textbook of Old Age Psychiatry*, it is the onset of multiple health problems in the elderly, rather than their age, that is bringing on the depression. In fact, the studies indicate that the prevalence of depression remains fairly much the same across the lifespan, although certain symptoms of depression are reported more often by elderly people than by those much younger. For example, older people with depression are more concerned with their physical ailments, and report less sadness than younger people with depression.

Perhaps this latter quality of the aged - to be more content, less sad - is the end result of many years of letting go. We cannot cling so ardently to the belief that we are this body when every falter in the step and loosening of the skin that comes with advancing years reminds us that we cannot be this degenerating form; subconsciously we realise that, "'I' have been observing this decline over the years, but 'I' am not changing."

As the wise Baba Ram Dass has written:

> *The sadness we often experience later in life may be just part of the Soul's evolution. Perhaps this depression is part of what Saint John calls the 'dark night of the Soul', in which the Ego experiences a kind of death in order to allow the Soul to be born into its own full Awareness.*

The presence of depression as a psychiatric disorder in the elderly may not always be easy to identify, particularly when the person's main reason for seeking medical assistance is to deal with their physical problems. Further, someone could be depressed, while at the same time having some other psychiatric disorder – whether they are depressed because of having the battle with their psychosis, or whether the two are coexisting, is often difficult to say. For these reasons, deciding when and how to medicate for depression is seldom straightforward.

Apart from medication – which of course can often make life a lot easier for the person who is caught up in the black fog of despair, self-doubt and negativity – what else can we as compassionate carers do to be of assistance to a depressed person in our care? As discussed in the previous chapter, the first step is to allow ourselves, to the extent that we are able, to empathically feel their pain, confusion and self-doubt, to feel their darkness within ourselves. This requires a degree of courage, until we are well-practised in feeling the pain while at the same time surrounding and saturating it with Love. There is a beautiful, yet powerful saying about making use of our depression as an impulse towards our inner delight. It says, "The stars shine brightest on the darkest night."

Essentially what we are saying is that, to the degree that we can utilise our own darkness as an opportunity to connect with our inner Love, joy and light, we will be able to silently convey (through our mirror neurons and the electromagnetic emanations from our heart) this inner wisdom to the one who is suffering.

The Human Values philosophy underlying the material in this Handbook is that all of our disturbing emotions – whether they be pain, sorrow, anger, envy or loneliness - are but impulses towards union with our higher Self, with the Love that saturates every one of our body's cells and all of the neurons in the brain. That is, we are proposing that depression has a purpose – as does sadness, annoyance and any other negative feeling – and that is: to prompt us to turn towards our inner ocean of delight, again and again, trusting that our darkness will make it easier for us to see a light not seen before. Some do this by turning towards their religion or to spirituality, prayer, affirmations or one of the fine arts; others use the loving-kindness meditation and other practices that we've introduced in these pages.

This is not to say that we can be certain of alleviating another's depression, but we can play a major role in bringing some light into a very dark room. Even the unspoken conviction, that within the depressed person there lies a limitless source of joy and contentment, will be of help to them. We can support such an assertion within ourselves by remembering that, regardless of how thick and heavy are the clouds that cover the sky, the sun remains shining in all of its splendour behind the very thick veil.

Relating in this way to the Sun in the one we are caring for, while at the same time feeling their 'clouds' as if we were in their shoes, shines a light for the lost one to see by; it gives hope and meaning where despair and confusion might reign.

For the convenience of the reader, we have listed in Appendix 2 the range of depression-based behaviours, and also some intervention strategies based largely on material covered in this Handbook. These are applicable more to residential aged care facilities, although many can be considered for use in the elderly person's home environment.

Although anxiety disorders are common among older people, there has been little research in this area compared to the attention given to other mental health problems afflicting the aged. Phobias and generalised anxiety (always anxious) are the two most common anxiety disorders in the aged. Those who endured the Second World War and the Holocaust as children and young adults are now well into old age, and many of them have been diagnosed with post-traumatic stress disorder (PTSD).

For the convenience of the reader, we have listed in Appendix 2 the range of anxiety-based behaviours and interventions relevant for those residing in aged care facilities. Most of the information is also useful for those elderly people being cared for in the home setting.

In addition to the range of interventions available to us, including medication, what else can we as compassionate carers do to be of assistance to an anxious person in our care? From the standpoint of the Human Values philosophy, the first step is to aim towards dispelling all of our own anxieties, big and small, and becoming lovingly fearless in how we live our lives. The point in doing this is that there develops within us a firm foundation of serenity and fearlessness, and this (again through our mirror neurons and the electromagnetic emanations from our heart) is very calming for the anxious or fear-filled person. Of course, this is a lifetime's task, but the rewards along the way, both for ourselves and for the ones we are caring for, are great indeed.

The Human Values of Love, Peace and Truth are the antidotes for all fears and anxieties. There is a saying in the Holy Bible: 'Perfect love casts out all fear'. And there is another saying in the profound book, *A Course in Miracles*, which says, in effect, 'There are only two emotions, Love and fear, and fear is but the shadow of Love'.

The image of light and dark explains both sayings very well. When we bring light into a darkened room, the darkness readily disappears. In the same way, when the heart opens in unconditional love for all, it is not possible for anxiety and fear to remain. Further, the analogy of the shadow tells us that, when we feel frightened or anxious, there is something in our beliefs, attitudes, hopes or expectations that is closing our heart – hence the advice in the *Course* that fear is the shadow of Love.

In the world of light and darkness, all shadows are caused by something blocking a light. Also, all shadows point back towards a light; that is, our anxiety and fear are telling us that a deeper and sweeter level of love is close by. In the same way as the discomfort of the stranded fish drives it to find water as soon as possible, our fear and anxiety can be used to impel us to be more forgiving, more loving, less judgmental, more patient and understanding.

As we have done for Love, an in-depth reflection on the Human Values of Peace and Truth will give further understanding of how our own fears and anxiety can be alleviated. We will leave it to those inspired by this approach to conduct that search for themselves. Such an exploration is certainly worthwhile, leading to more freedom in how we live, and to the joy in witnessing how our calm presence can be of real help to the anxious and fearful ones in our care.

Dementia

What follows is a very brief synopsis of what is presently known about dementia.

Dementia is not a single specific disease. It is an umbrella term describing a syndrome associated with more than 100 different diseases that are characterised by the impairment of brain functions, including language, memory, perception, personality and cognitive skill. Although the type and severity of symptoms and their pattern of development varies with the type of dementia, it is usually of gradual onset, progressive in nature and irreversible.

The World Health Organisation regards dementia as a global epidemic. The number of people with dementia worldwide in 2015 was estimated to be nearly 48 million, and is predicted to reach 135 million in 2050, the increase mainly due to the population living much longer, particularly in the non-rich countries.

The need for support from a caregiver often starts early in the dementia journey and intensifies as the illness progresses over time. There is a large research literature on the extent of the strain that caregivers experience, weighed down with physical, psychological and economic burdens.

The most common types of dementia are Alzheimer's disease, vascular dementia, dementia with Lewy bodies, and frontotemporal dementia (which includes Pick disease). We will give a little information about each one.

Description of the most common types of dementia

Alzheimer's disease is the most common type of dementia, accounting for about 50% to 75% of dementia cases worldwide. It is characterised by short-term memory loss, apathy and depression in the early stages. Onset is gradual and decline is progressive. This form is most common among older people with dementia, particularly among women.

Vascular dementia is generally considered to be the second most common type of dementia, with about 20% to 30% of dementia cases thought to be of this type. It is caused by cerebrovascular conditions (for example, stroke). Symptoms in the early stages are similar to Alzheimer's disease, but memory loss is not as great and mood fluctuations are more prominent. Physical frailty is also evident. Onset can be sudden. The course of the disease is less predictable than Alzheimer's disease, with decline more likely to be stepwise.

Frontotemporal dementia is thought to account for about 5% to 10% of cases and is relatively more common in males with a younger onset of dementia. Early symptoms include personality and mood changes, disinhibition and language difficulties.

Dementia with Lewy bodies accounts for up to 5% of cases and is associated with the development of abnormal cells, called Lewy bodies, in the brain.

Characteristic symptoms include marked fluctuation in cognitive ability and visual hallucinations, as well as symptoms similar to Parkinson's disease (for example, tremor and rigidity). Progression tends to be more rapid than Alzheimer's disease.

(Source: Alzheimer's Disease International 2009; Draper, 2011; Seeher et al. 2011)

Risk and Protective Factors for Dementia

What causes dementia is still being investigated. The disease is known to begin laying down markers up to 80 years before the symptoms become a serious problem. Dementia is the end stage of the disease when the brain has become sufficiently damaged for its function to be significantly affected.

Although there is no certifiable way of preventing dementia, a large body of research studies have delved into environmental factors that we should act on so as to lower the risk, or at least delay the onset, of the disease. However, these identifiable risk and protective factors are more like probabilities than certainties. Let us touch on the risk factors first.

The main risk factor for most types of dementia is advancing age. The research studies are consistent in saying that the prevalence of dementia appears to increase exponentially with age from about 65 years, doubling every 5 or 6 years. Lifestyle factors that seem to increase the risk of dementia include smoking, midlife obesity, physical inactivity, low education or cognitive inactivity, depression and midlife hypertension. Some of these overlap with the elements of healthy living identified by international research studies as being likely to prevent or delay the onset of Alzheimer's and other dementias.

Alzheimer's and other dementias are complex diseases with multiple risk factors. Some, like our age and genetics, are outside our control. But many others are within our sphere of influence. And these factors can be quite powerful when it comes to our brain health. By identifying and controlling our personal risk and preventative factors, we can maximize our chances of lifelong brain health and take effective steps to preserve our cognitive abilities.

Reviews of the research studies indicate that the components of a brain-healthy, Alzheimer's-prevention lifestyle are:

1. Regular physical activity
2. Healthy diet
3. Ongoing intellectual stimulation
4. Leisure/social activities
5. Higher education
6. Quality sleep
7. Stress management

In Chapter 3 we discussed the Healthy Mind Platter as developed by Daniel Siegel, David Rock and their colleagues in 2011, the elements of which are in accord with the above lifestyle factors.

There are numerous other possible protective factors for which evidence is less conclusive, including intake of omega-3 fatty acids, and use of cholesterol-lowering medications, nonsteroidal anti-inflammatory medications and aspirin.

Typical Behavioural and Psychological Symptoms of Dementia

Regardless of its etiology, dementia is a clinical syndrome that expresses itself in three areas: cognitive deficits, psychiatric and behavioural disturbance, and difficulties in carrying out daily functions. In 1996, the International Psychogeriatric Association convened a consensus conference on the behavioural disturbances in dementia. The consensus group made this statement:

The term behavioural disturbances should be replaced by the term BPSD (Behavioural and Psychological Symptoms of Dementia), defined as symptoms of disturbed perception, thought content, mood or behaviour that frequently occur in patients with dementia.

In *The Best Practice Guideline for Accommodating and Managing Behavioural and Psychological Symptoms of Dementia in Residential Care (the guideline)* published in 2012, the range of behavioural and psychological symptoms of dementia (BPSD) include the following:

- ◇ Aggression
- ◇ Agitation, and/or restlessness
- ◇ Screaming
- ◇ Pacing and repetitive motor activity
- ◇ Anxiety
- ◇ Depression
- ◇ Psychosis (delusions and hallucinations)
- ◇ Repetitive vocalization, cursing and swearing
- ◇ Sleep disturbance
- ◇ Shadowing (following the carer closely)
- ◇ Sundowning (state of agitation, confusion, anxiety and aggressiveness in late afternoon, in the evening, or at night)
- ◇ Wandering
- ◇ Hoarding

For these and other disturbing behaviours we have included in Appendix 2 a more comprehensive list of disturbed behaviour and possible interventions that may be able to help the troubled person find physical comfort and peace of mind.

Many reading this chapter will be full-time carers for a loved one at home, or a professional caregiver visiting homes, or working in a residential aged care facility. The fact that you choose to do this is an inspiration to all of us, for you are the ones at the forefront of change. It is only in recent decades that dementia and other age-related diseases have come into prominence because of our increasing longevity. Often without sufficient physical and emotional support – particularly the elderly caring for the elderly at home – somehow you give of yourself again and again, for the sake of those in your care. We trust that what we have touched on in this chapter can be of some help in understanding and managing the challenges confronting you every day.

Opportunities to find deeper powers within ourselves come when life seems most challenging.

Joseph Campbell

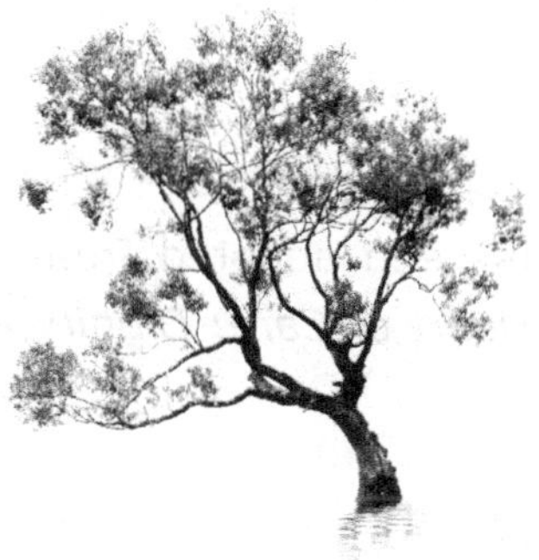

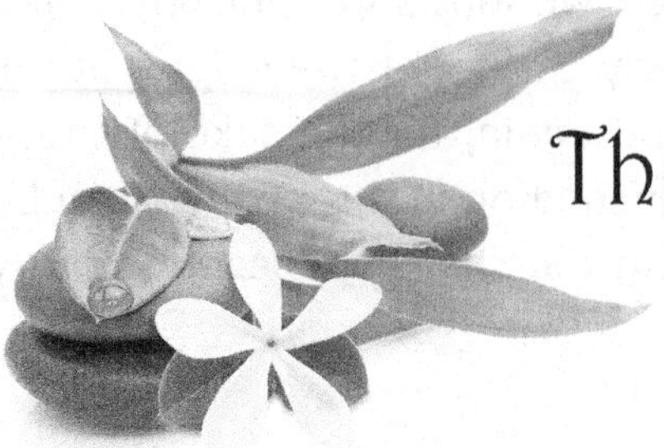

The Practice

EXERCISE TO UNDERSTAND
BEING A PERSON WITH DEMENTIA

To fully understand the challenges and stresses a person with dementia is facing, we need to walk in their shoes. This will help us to understand their specific needs and the positive steps we can take to support them.

<u>Exercise:</u>
If You Had Dementia

The following exercise has been adapted from *Insight into Dementia* by Rosemary Hurtley in *The Heart of Care: Dignity in Action* by Amanda Waring, 2012.

How can I do this exercise?

◇ Spend 5 to 10 mins. on each section of this exercise, imagining yourself in that condition, and write down what your experience was like – perhaps what you felt, what came into your mind, and any physical reactions you may have observed.

◇ If you had dementia you would probably have problems with ideas, words, speech and possibly hearing, as well as repeating yourself. You would suffer from confusion of people, time or place; have difficulties in instigating and continuing a conversation; and trouble with making decisions, often forgetting mid-flow what is being talked about. You would find yourself dwelling in the past and over-reaching. The carers who look after you need patience and reassurance to be able to meet you in your present or Now, along your own spectrum of 'time travel'.

◇ If you had dementia you would experience mood swings. So those who care for you need to be aware of the nuances of your behaviour and to identify if you are being influenced by physical pain or emotional pain or both.

◇ If you had dementia you would experience increasing problems understanding what is being said to you and what is going on around you. You may find it very difficult to communicate with others and may gradually lose your speech or cry out from time to time. Those caring for you need to remember that verbal language is only one way of communicating; they need to take time to observe your expressions and body language, which will provide them with clues as to how you are feeling.

◇ If you had dementia you would possibly also have a visual or hearing impairment, and so be frustrated at experiencing further barriers. You would feel an isolation due to a lack of awareness of your environment, which could lead to you having a fear of falling or of having accidents. You would have an all-pervading sense of anxiety. You would need carers to reach you, support and reassure you as you feel yourself suffering from withdrawal, having less opportunity for participation, and reduced involvement in all activities. You would need carers to give emotional and practical support to retain your interests within your capabilities, to include you in positive social encounters, and to provide sufficient activity choices and meaningful roles.

◇ If you had dementia, could you see why your behaviour may be uncooperative, and wouldn't you rather your carer understood the underlying reasons rather than force medication on you?

May I be an island for those who yearn for landfall,
And a lamp for those who long for light;
For those who need a resting place, a bed;
For all who need a servant, may I be their help.

May I be the wishing jewel, the vase of plenty,
A word of power and the supreme remedy,
May I be the tree of miracles,
And for every being the cow of abundance.

Like the earth and the pervading elements,
Enduring as the sky itself endures,
For boundless multitudes of living beings,
May I be their ground and sustenance.

Shantideva

Chapter 15

Nurturing the Wellbeing of the Caregiver

Have good trust in yourself -
not in the one that you think you should be,
but in the one that you are.

Maezumi Roshi

Across the international research spectrum, it has been found that the mental and emotional strain on caregivers for the aged, whether employed in residential aged care facilities, or caring for a loved one at home, can become intolerable. The challenge for those who are 'on duty' for the 24 hours in every day in their own home, usually alone except for all-too-brief respite periods, is particularly difficult, sometimes unbearable. For the residential care professionals, although they have their rest periods away from the work situation, the arduousness of their role has much to do with being face-to-face with so many living examples of how diseases of the brain and nervous system can wreak havoc in the lives of so many once-vibrant, active and strong personalities. How can the selfless, compassionate caregiver find peace of mind in such demanding circumstances?

It is our belief and understanding – derived from the ancient wisdom that unites all of the major religions – that within each one of us lies a treasure of unbounded proportions and inestimable value. Through times of joy and sadness, harmony and discord, enchantment and disillusionment, we search together for the Holy Grail, that feeling of authentic happiness and wellbeing that is ever-lasting and ever-present.

We yearn always to reach this elusive goal, this feeling of loving Oneness, this mutual joy, at this time and in these circumstances. We yearn for this deep level of shared love, because deep down we sense that we are Love. We are looking for our true Self, that Self which is common to us all, which is Love. And we strive to manifest in ourselves all of the other noble human virtues because we intuitively know that they are our birthright. Nobody wants to feel unloved, because lack of love is not our natural state; and we do not want to feel agitated, because equanimity is the crown we are born to wear, and the same applies to every positive feeling, virtue and activity.

In the same way that the fish stranded on the rock will do whatever it can to return to the water where it belongs, any discomfort or disharmony in our life and relationships prompts us to renew our search for our natural state of love, peace and joy.

However, whereas the fish knows without any doubt where the life-saving water lies, many of us are completely unaware that what we are looking and striving for already lies deep within us. Not realising (or forgetting) this, we always look outside of ourselves for relief to come.

We have been looking in the wrong place for our love, calm, beauty and delight, perhaps ever since humans first walked the earth, as illustrated by St Augustine of Hippo (354-430 AD) when he wrote in his *Confessions* these words of celebration and yearning:

> *Late have I loved you,*
> *O Beauty so ancient and so new;*
> *late have I loved you!*

You were within me, but I was outside,
and it was there that I searched for you.

It is not always easy, in the role of the compassionate caregiver, to see beauty, love and light in the ones we are tending to, and in the environment in which our dedicated service takes place. Sometimes exhausted, at other times overwhelmed by the sheer immensity of the task before us, we need to remind ourselves that the sun is always shining behind the clouds, and that a hidden fire lies waiting inside the unburnt log of wood. At our lowest, when it all seems too much, it is sometimes helpful to remember that our Soul, our higher Self, is always trying to get our attention, to call us Home and that it can use the sudden inrush of acceptance, humility and peace to do this, or it can arrange for the body to give us powerful signals commanding us to slow down, be present, give thanks, watch the breath, earnestly pray, smile, chant our mantra, repeat our affirmation or just let go in humility. "Yes. Yes. I let go. I let go. Do with me as Thou wilt."

Whatever our condition, whatever the situation, we can profit by giving credence to the age-old knowledge that we are, in Truth, every one of the noble virtues; we are the five Human Values of Love, Truth, Peace, Right Conduct and Non-violence, in their pristine form; and by reasoning that, if we are the light, we cannot be the dark. Each one of our fears, resentments, waves of helplessness, and all else that we want to end, are not who we truly are, and they make us yearn even more for the peace, love, beauty, joy and light that is our birthright.

Most of us would agree from our own experience that, if we could live every moment of our lives feeling a peace beyond compare, one that was unaffected by whatever happens to us, we would have discovered a level of happiness that we all yearn for. Surely unruffled equanimity and contentment – a deep abiding peace – is the most priceless possession we could ever have. Imagine if we learned how to feel so peaceful, regardless of external events, regardless of how unfair or impossible life seems to be.

Without a doubt we would be very happy, with a state of wellbeing that eludes almost everybody.

Imagine if we felt a great warmth and affection for everyone at work, in the family and in the community; and if we expressed our feelings of kindness and compassion for others by always being on the lookout for ways to offer help in some way to those in need. And imagine that we knew without a doubt that a vast, limitless ocean of perfect Love already lay within us, independent of the love that may or may not be directed towards us by others. Surely we too would be radiating a level of unalloyed happiness that would light up the lives of all who come near us.

Strategies to nurture the wellbeing of the caregiver

As you can see throughout the Handbook, the words above represent the philosophy underlying a Human Values approach to living, growing, working, aging and passing over. For those who can accept it, the purpose and meaning of life arising out of such attitudes are forever bearing fruit. They lay a solid foundation for the compassionate caregiver to explore and apply a wide range of stress-reducing and heart-opening self-help techniques for rediscovering our Peaceful Mind, Open Heart.

In Chapter 4 we touched on the five foundations for experiencing authentic happiness and wellbeing, and included exercises for cultivating positivity in our life.

Based on the many practices in different chapters of this Handbook, the following strategies for nurturing the carers' wellbeing have been developed:

1. Applying Peaceful Mind, Open Heart throughout our daily activities.

If we want to find and follow the pathway to Peaceful Mind, Open Heart, we have only to observe a one-year-old baby to remember what to do. We were babies once, and the approach that we followed intuitively then was to make use of every available moment to observe, explore, love and to learn. As it was then, so it is now. Every activity, every pause, every struggle and every interaction with others is a unique and potent opportunity for us to: practise the Carer's Code of Conduct; be mindfully aware by watching our Words, Actions, Thoughts, Character and Heart (WATCH); become more sensitive and skilled in our loving, dutiful roles; remember that we are not the body, but rather an unchanging Spirit residing for a while in an ever-aging body; use the imagination for exploring ageless Truths such as 'I am the movie, not the screen' or 'I am a wave on an endless sea, an inseparable part of the sea'; and to make good use of the truism that, if everyone is a mirror for us to see our preferences and prejudices, when we have Peaceful Mind, Open Heart we will see only beauty in all whom we meet.

There are many techniques we can use to find and stay on the Path. Some suggestions for doing this are included in:

> *A Guideline for Peaceful Mind, Open Heart throughout our daily activities*, in Appendix 1 of this Handbook.

2. Managing emotions and developing resilience

When we feel stressed, overwhelmed, anxious, angry or depressed in our struggle to care for others in a respectful and committed way, it can seem that there is no solution, no way out of a demanding and difficult situation. At such times it can be useful to recall the simple refrain:

It matters not which way the wind blows,
it is how we set our sails.

To appreciate the metaphor, we can picture a boat sailing along parallel to a rocky shore. It does not matter to the sailor whether the wind is blowing towards or away from the shore. Either way, the sails can be adjusted so that the wind keeps moving the boat along in the desired direction. In the same way, we can regard our emotions (any emotions, whether positive or negative) as we do the wind. The negative ones are threatening to blow us towards self-destruction, while the positive ones appear to make life easier but can still get us lost in the open sea. It is what we do with our mind (the sails) that matters – how we think.

If we keep our mind focussed on our goal of Peaceful Mind, Open Heart, we can use the power of emotion to take us there. When disturbing feelings come, we must ensure that our thinking does not add power to this 'wind' to close our heart and destroy our peace of mind. Rather, we can hold onto thoughts that harness the power of our emotions to open our heart and foster peace of mind. As an example of this, following a Buddhist inclination, we are advised:

When you are feeling bad,
Practise compassion and loving-kindness.
When you are feeling good,
Practise compassion and loving-kindness.

The image of the wind and the sailing boat is but one of many metaphors and guidances for learning how to regulate our emotions. Without developing this skill, we remain at the mercy of whatever our thoughts and feelings happen to be. But of course it takes resilience to be able to insist on being master of the mind instead of its slave. That is, we can assert our higher Self by choosing what to think, rather than allowing old patterns of thinking to remain.

There are many techniques for regulating our emotions and developing the necessary resilience to be able to do so.

Some suggestions for doing this include:

◇ Exercises for self-awareness and self-regulation
(All exercises in Chapter 3)

3. Managing levels of stress

Not too long ago we listened to the spiritual teacher Sathya Sai Baba talking about what we generally refer to as stress. He said something like:

All of the troubles in the world are caused by ego and attachment;
and the solution to all of the world's problems
are humility and detachment.

According to our understanding, *ego* is the delusion or incorrect thinking that we are this transient body, rather than its immortal resident, and that we are the ones doing everything. Consequently, we feel bad if we try and then find that we can't control events, and we feel good when we succeed and think that we have achieved something. *Humility* is knowing that everything is being done through us; that we are like a flute being played by the master; and that our contribution is to ensure that, like the flute, we are straight and hollow.

Again, according to our understanding, *attachment* is what we want and desire. Using the analogy of electricity: if our hand gets too close to the live electric wire, our fist closes around it; we cannot let go and suffer greatly. Similarly, if we get too close to (identify with) our thoughts, feelings, our body, desires, actions, sensations, memory and ability to discriminate, we become attached to them, unable to let go, so that we are dominated by them, enslaved by them. *Detachment* is not getting too close to the wire. It means knowing that we are not any of the above (thoughts, feelings, etc.), and knowing that everything we seek or desire (e.g. happiness, love, etc.) is already within us.

So when we feel stressed, it can be helpful to remember that, because we are observing the stress, we know that we are not the stress; and that we are the screen, untouched by the movie about stress projected onto our surface. And we might remind ourselves that 'Everything is being done through me', and any of the other de-stressing methods described throughout the Handbook.

Some suggestions for exploring these possibilities include:

◇ Exercises for the blossoming of human excellence in the brain (All exercises in Chapter 5)
◇ Exercises to regulate the mind and the brain (All exercises in Chapter 6)
◇ Exercises for cultivating heart-intelligence (All exercises in Chapter 7)
◇ Exercises for growing the brain (All exercises in Chapter 9)

4. Living in the present moment

News about the benefits of mindfulness is now reaching into all segments of society. Even top companies such as Google and IBM have created their own downloadable guided-mindfulness exercises for all of their employees to use. After thousands of years of ignoring the Treasure lying within our grasp, modern society is now recognising that focussing on what is happening right now, in this present moment, from moment to moment, without expectation or judgment, brings not only peace of mind, an opening of the heart, but also increased clarity, concentration and creativity.

There are many exercises for developing mindful awareness, for living in the present moment. Some suggestions include:

◇ Exercises for mindful awareness
(All exercises in Chapter 11)
◇ Exercises for living mindfully
(All exercises in Chapter 12)

5. Enhancing positivity in our life

After a century of focussing on what was wrong with people, with what we are lacking, modern psychology realised that it was more effective to increase the light source rather than try to analyse the darkness. And so positive psychology was born, with its emphasis upon expressing gratitude for great and small, identifying and utilising our character strengths, using the imagination to send loving-kindness and other noble feelings to others, and so much more.

As compassionate carers, it helps to remind ourselves that ours is a noble cause. We are engaged in the highest form of unconditional loving , putting the care and comfort of others before our own. There are clear indications that the example being set by such selfless, loving service is reawakening an interest in and respect for the elderly, who once gave so much to build this modern society that we now enjoy.

There are a number of simple methods that can be used to enhance positivity in our life.

Some suggestions for doing this include:

◇ Exercises to cultivate positivity in our life
(All exercises in Chapter 4)

◇ Exercises for rejuvenating the power of gratitude
(All exercises in Chapter 8)
◇ Exercises for acknowledging the gift of caring
(All exercises in Chapters 13 and 14)

6. Connecting with our true Nature

As has been noted earlier, many wise ones throughout history have sought to convince the blind that a sun does exist in the sky - that a vast treasure of wisdom, joy, love and power lies within us, like fire hidden inside wood; like the perfect form lying within the rough block of stone awaiting to be revealed by the chiselling of the sculptor. Saint Francis of Assisi said, "What you are looking for, is what is looking." That is, we seek to defuse stress and find peace, because we are Peace. And we seek to be loved, because we are Love. In everything we do, think, say and feel, we are looking for that Pathway that will lead us Home, to rediscover our true Self. We are the only part of Nature that is not completely and constantly in touch with its true essence. The nature of fire is to burn and so give off warmth and light - and that is what it does. The nature of water is to quench thirst, nurture growth, and to be useful when heated - and again, that is what water does. The wise ones have told us, using so many metaphors, reasoning and illustrations, that our true nature is love and wisdom, and that our innate yearning and purpose in life is to rediscover these Treasures within, and to share them with others.

Throughout the Handbook we have referred to our five universal Human Values of Love, Truth, Peace, Right Conduct and Non-violence, manifesting as Peaceful Mind, Open Heart. There are a thousand pathways to the summit of the mountain. Some suggestions that you might like to explore include:

◇ Exercises for rediscovering our five innate Human Values
(All exercises in Chapter 2)

- ◇ Exercises to reveal the unchanging Self
  (All exercises in Chapter 10)
- ◇ Exercises to connect with our true nature
  (All exercises in Chapter 15)

7. Creating and engaging in regular, planned events that are pleasurable and relaxing

These occassions offer us an opportunity for self-renewal. Some of us will enjoy watching the sunrise, tending the garden, walking on the beach, riding a bicycle, visiting sacred sites, watching a good movie, and so on. Whatever it is, it is important that we create opportunities that will allow the brain and nervous system to re-balance and rest by spending time away from the demands of our responsibilities. Until we have rediscoverd the full measure of the inner Treasure awaiting us, we will need to enjoy the external world, giving thanks for the multitude of gifts that are pouring into our life constantly.

8. Building a support system

As with all living things, we gravitate naturally towards the company of those whose life and behaviour reflect back to us the best of what we are seeking in ourselves. Not only that, we recognise that a clear picture of the one mountain of Truth comes when we spend time with others who are seeing another side of things. This helps us broaden our perspective so that we can have different ways of looking at the same issue, thereby getting us out of our singular viewpoint which may have been hampering our journey towards authentic happiness and wellbeing.

Some suggestions for opening doors so that others can enrich our lives by their wise and loving presence include:

- ◇ Connecting with family, friends, and other caregivers
- ◇ Spending time with your support network

9. Engaging in an ongoing learning task

The continuation of learning throughout life has the benefits of enhancing our self-esteem, encouraging social interaction and a more active life.

Fieldwork studies indicate that participation in lifelong learning can play a major role in nurturing our sense of wellbeing and also developing the resilience to be able to travel unhindered through the ups and downs of life. These positive effects appear to grow in tandem with increases in self-esteem, self-efficacy, a sense of purpose and hope, competencies and social interaction.

Nurturing the wellbeing of the compassionate caregiver is important not only because their physical, psychological, social, educational and spiritual gifts are so vital and precious for the one in care; and not only so they can continue their truly selfless service. Such care for the caregiver is also for other reasons as well, an important one of which can be expressed as:

> To the extent that we can find ways of restoring our own inner calm, and strengthening open-heartedness and joy in living, this will have a potent effect upon all of those less-fortunate ones we are caring for. We know from our own experience that we feel more peaceful, almost immediately, in the presence of one who is in touch with a deep ocean of serenity within themselves. And, regardless of our mood and troubles, we open one of the doors into our own inner Treasure House of Love when a truly compassionate person talks with us, cares for us, and is so gentle and kind to us.

The song that the compassionate carer sings resonates with the song yet to be sung by others. And the dance that we do can inspire another to allow the dance to be danced through them. For this reason too, let us nurture the wellbeing of the caregiver.

Let me, O let me bathe my soul
in colours; let me swallow the sunset
and drink the rainbow.

Kahlil Gibran

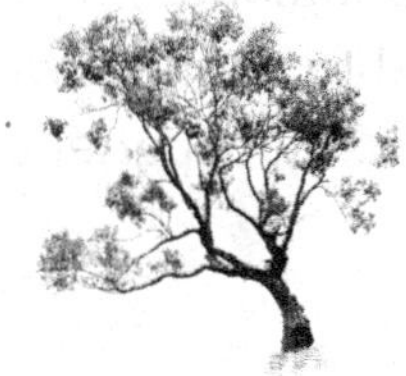

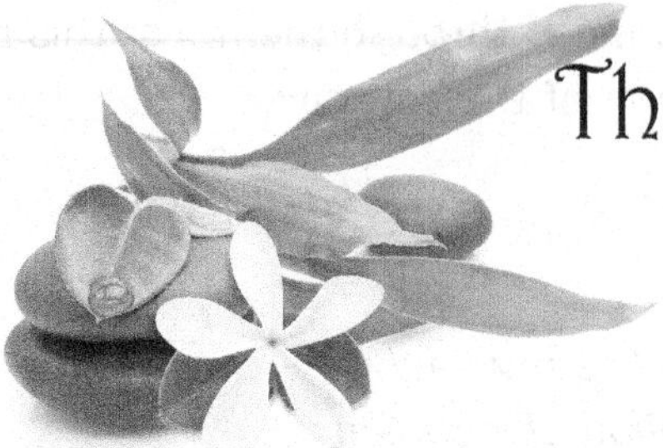

The Practice

EXERCISES TO CONNECT WITH OUR TRUE SELF

Exercise 1:
Treasuring Beauty

The following exercise will have maximum effect if you endeavour to relive vividly the events you are asked to connect with and if you do so with all of your senses, as if you were actually experiencing them.

How can I do this exercise?

- ◇ Start by recollecting several moments of beauty, one by one. They may include the beauty of Nature, of a relationship, of growth, of understanding, and so on. The choice is yours. Feel their special effect upon you, as fully as you can.
- ◇ Take your time in relishing these moments; let them sink into you so that you can assimilate them, realize how valuable they are and treasure them. Remind yourself that this beauty is always within you.
- ◇ Now take some time to allow a sense of openness within you to grow – an openness to the totality of your being. Allow yourself to realise the depth of your sensitivity, and of the vibrant interest that you have in the presence of beauty in everyone and everything.

While exploring beauty in its many appearances, we may have the privileged experience of connecting with it, independently of any form. This is what Plato described as the beauty which 'neither waxes nor wanes'; it is St Augustine's 'Beauty so ancient and so new'; Shelley's 'Spirit of Beauty'. These are not just poetical metaphors. They are actual psychological experiences having a profound impact on those who are experiencing them. Describing this kind of contact with the ineffable, one person writes:

I was looking at a peach tree in blossom, and then I suddenly felt that it was not just the tree that was beautiful, but living beauty seemed to be coming through it, and it was in touch with me. It was an intensely personal contact, and it was like some being was communicating with me in a wordless way. It was like meeting some very, very special person who had an extraordinary effect on me.

This entity, I felt, was seeking at all times to express itself through the activity of innumerable forms of life – through nature, as with a flower or a spider weaving a web, or through a human being creating a work of art – so that the same life could express itself through me. It was a wonderful moment. I experienced great strength in my body, and I was flooded by an overwhelming sense of harmony. In a flash, countless aspects of beauty were revealed to me which I had never realized before.

◇ Spend 5 to 10 minutes contemplating on what it would be like to have this experience. Write about one of your own experiences of treasuring beauty, and your understanding of it all.

Exercise 2:

The Temple of Silence

This exercise is to provide an experience of the imagination leading us into those inner realms of purity, reverence and silence that are ever-present, and inviting us always to journey within so we can merge with our higher Self, with the Oneness that we truly are.

How can I do this exercise?

- ◊ Imagine a hill covered with greenery. A path leads to the top, where you can see the Temple of Silence. Using your imagination, allow the shape of the Temple to represent your higher Self: noble, harmonious, and radiant.
- ◊ Imagine that it is a spring morning, sunny and pleasantly warm. Notice how you are dressed. Become conscious of your body ascending the path, and feel the contact of your feet with the ground. Feel the breeze on your cheeks. Look around you at the trees and the bushes, the grass, and the wildflowers as you go up the hill.
- ◊ Imagine that you are now approaching the top of the hill. Ageless stillness pervades the atmosphere of the Temple of Silence. No word has even been uttered here. You are close to its big wooden door. See your hands on them and feel the wood. Before opening the door, know that when you do so, you will be surrounded by silence.
- ◊ Imagine that you enter the Temple. You feel the atmosphere of stillness and peace all around you. You walk forward into the silence, looking about you as you go. You see a big, luminous dome. Its luminosity not only comes from the rays of the sun, but also seems to spring from within and to be concentrated in an area of radiance just in front of you.
- ◊ Imagine that you enter this luminous silence and feel absorbed by it. Peaceful beams of warm, gentle and soothing light are enveloping you. Let this luminous silence pervade you. Feel it flowing through your veins and permeating every cell in your body.

◇ Imagine that you remain in this luminous silence for two or three minutes, very alert and present in the moment. During this time, listen to the silence. Silence is a living quality; it is not just the mere absence of sounds.

◇ Imagine that you slowly leave the area of radiance, walk back through the Temple and out through the doors. Outside, open yourself to the impact of the springtime; feel its gentle breeze once more on your cheeks, and listen to the singing of the birds.

Exercise 3:
Looking Inside for Happiness

Each of us, the whole world over, yearns for two boons, two gifts, to accompany us through every stage of our life. They are: the attainment of joy, and escape from sorrow. These two are inextricably linked.

We spend most of our time searching for ways to be happy, because we know with a subliminal, unspoken certainty that lasting peace and joy are rightfully ours. We find it hard to settle for less.

However, forgetting that this vast ocean of happiness already lies waiting within, our search misleads our attention away from our true Self, towards temporary worldly delights. We are like the man who is standing knee-deep in a pure, flowing stream, holding out his cup, begging for a little water to quench his thirst.

The challenge is to develop the habit of finding our ever-present, inner contentment well before those closing years when the external sources of delight might be increasingly denied to us by our destiny. Let us spend some time looking within for our Treasure.

How can I do this exercise?

- ◇ You might like to begin by repeating the following affirmation as often as you can, reflecting on each part:

  Within me is pure, lasting, unsullied happiness.
  Within me is a vast, limitless ocean of nectar divine.
  I seek it. I find it. I find it.

- ◇ If you do this several times a day for a few weeks, you will start to believe that it is Truth; then you'll begin to catch glimpses of a happiness never known before.

Should you really open your eyes and see,
you would behold your image in all images.
And should you open your ears and listen,
you would hear your own voice in all voices.

Kahlil Gibran

Epilogue

Where the Road Ends

I had travelled a long
and hard dusty road,
strewn with leftovers
from hopes and dreams
and wants and dislikes,
hoping to find somewhere
the elixir that would
ease the ache in my heart,
or a song that would
lift me to another plane
above this one that
sang only of loneliness,
sorrow, fear and pain.

My horse was now lame,
the water bag empty,
the flowers all wilted or died,
and the friends I once knew
couldn't reach me anymore,
for I was lost somewhere,
with a mind chasing thoughts
that always eluded me
like butterflies in the sun.

"Do I know you?
I might have known someone
who reminds me of you,
but nothing stays in my mind
long enough for me to know."

So in my loneliness and pain,
I waited long outside
this door that was closed,
knocking to see if anyone
still lives somewhere
deep in this heart of mine.

I knew what I needed
but couldn't find any words,
not one little raindrop
from the storm that was inside.

And then one day there came
a Soul just like me,
one who had left behind
the secure comfort of mind
to enter that place of no change,
that place in the heart
where all beings reside.

I was knocking on the door
and it opened from inside,
and there was this Soul,
the one who had left
all of the mind behind.

Oh, the joy and the love
that enveloped me then,
as Soul led me inside
and everyone was there.

It was so good to know
that really nothing had changed,
that 'I' was still 'I',
that 'I' was pure love,
as were all in that room,
that place in the heart
where all beings reside.

My horse is still lame,
the water bag dry,
the flowers all wilted or died,
but now I can fly
in an infinite sky,
and my tears of rejoicing
the only Treasure I need.

Of course I still wander off
and walk out through the door,
getting lost with the butterflies
always filling my mind.

Then the door somehow appears
and I knock on it once more
and Soul welcomes me in,
brings me in through the door.
"Where have you been?
I was looking for you.
It's so good that you've returned.
This heart's incomplete if you're not here."

There's one thing I'll say more
before this body fades.
I'll share with you now
what this mind did not know.

Where the road ends
is where it all began,
that place in the heart
where every being resides.

The gold did not change
when the bracelet was made,
nor did the potter's clay
when it was moulded and dried.

The journey we are on
gives the illusion of change,
of happiness and pain,
of good fortune and none,
of bodies that are born
that will grow old one day.

But we are the Changeless,
the One observing it all;
with Peaceful Mind
and Open Heart
forever guiding us Home.

APPENDIX 1

Integrating Peaceful Mind, Open Heart and Mindfulness Approaches into our Daily Routine: A Guideline for Compassionate Carers

1. Greeting the Day

You might like to look around you each morning before you get out of bed to meet the day, recognising the experience of coming out of sleep into conscious awareness, with a sense of gratitude. The feeling is more one of opening the heart to gratitude, rather than making a statement.

You could greet the day silently, or with words like, "Thank you, for another beautiful day." And you might like to add 3 or more things that you are grateful for, such as, "Thank you for (name) who is so kind to me. Thank you for all of the sounds that I can hear, and thank you for this work that I love doing," and so on, whatever is appropriate for you.

Greeting the day involves witnessing and participating in its arrival. Your expressions of gratitude open doors into your Peaceful Mind and Open Heart, so that your mood and behaviour are positively influenced all day long.

2. Practising Mindful Breathing

Allow a minimum time of 10 minutes every morning to practise mindful breathing.

After referring to Chapter 11 to select a preferred mindful awareness exercise, consider options for integrating a shortened form into different aspects of your morning routine. That is, look for opportunities to create mini Peaceful Mind, Open Heart exercises.

3. Breakfast

Whether it be a giving of thanks for food about to be shared, or having a sacred eating ritual, the blessing and partaking of food is one of the main ways in which we can express and embody our connection with all living things.

If you are at home and can be alone in the kitchen, prepare your meal mindfully, handling the food carefully and moving around the kitchen slowly. When you sit down to eat, just eat. Don't do anything else. Even the simplest food is a gift from so many plants and animals; even water and air are miracles we rarely think of.

Take one bite, paying attention to what is happening in your mouth, noticing the taste. Don't rush; take one bite at a time, noticing how the taste changes, how your teeth and tongue work ... Take your time. Be curious about your experience. When you are eating, take notice of how your body, mind and heart feel now, in this moment.

4. On the Way to Work

As you prepare to leave for work, notice how your body, mind and emotions are feeling. Are you calm and relaxed, or pressed for time and stressed about organising everything you need? If you live with other people, take a moment to reflect on your interactions. Were they fulfilling or unsettling? If you notice escalating emotions and recognise the possibility of impending conflict, pause and apply a mindfulness technique.

Giving our loved ones our full attention as we say goodbye and wish them a good day, is a great gift – for them and for us as well.

5. At Work

◇ STOP before you start

Reflecting on some of the shorter exercises in the Handbook, decide on what might be the first thing to do when you enter the work-place. You could use the STOP technique and then greet your colleagues and clients by acknowledging their presence and communicating a warm welcome.

Pace yourself realistically – with Peaceful Mind and Open Heart – especially if you have a few minutes between getting to work and the first task of interacting with others.

◇ Starting activities

The first step is to take a few slow, deep breaths to assess the situation, noticing what is happening, with a Peaceful Mind and Open Heart.

There are two strategies that can be applied at the beginning of any activity which can help your client engage in the activity with a Peaceful Mind and Open Heart:

- Reading aloud a wise saying, a poem or the lyrics from a special song. Pick the material that has uplifting virtues in it, and that resonates with your clients and the environment.

- Use a short mindful breathing exercise.

  You can instruct your clients to place their hands on their chest, noticing how the body is breathing, and listen to the sound of a musical note for one minute. You can use percussion instruments like the triangle or chime to make a simple reverberating sound.

◇ Throughout the day

At various times throughout the day, introduce a selection of short mini mindfulness practices: e.g. mindfulness of the breath, mindfulness of sounds, the STOP technique, Shift-and-Shine approach and Self-as-the-Observer (see Chapter 3).

◇ Concluding the day's work

Whenever possible at the end of the work day, part company with your colleagues and clients with a 'goodbye' that is grounded in a Peaceful Mind and Open Heart.

Allow time to acknowledge the positive behaviour and experiences that you have observed during the day. Communicate your appreciation to others with a Peaceful Mind and Open Heart that nurtures the feeling of Oneness.

6. Heading Home

Once you leave your work and exit the building, take a few deep breaths of the outside air and look up at the sky. Smell and listen to the environment around you, even if the odours and sounds aren't attractive. Mark the transition from work to home and consciously place yourself in your new environment with a Peaceful Mind and Open Heart.

When you get home, it is likely that you'll encounter only a few people, if any. Notice this difference and allow yourself time to adjust.

Personal time is important and healthy, whether we prefer to be alone or with others. Mindfulness has a role here too. It increases our sensitivity to noticing inner experiences and the outer environment, while shifting our attention into the present.

You might like to consider the following steps as preparation for sleep:

- ◇ Focus on your breathing. Take a few deep breaths.
- ◇ Review your experiences during the day, noticing distinct events and transitions, without judging what happened.
- ◇ Identify an experience about which you feel pleased with your involvement, and feel that pleasure again.
- ◇ Identify an experience about which you feel dissatisfied, and consider a more constructive approach for the next time.
- ◇ Notice that you are Here and Now.
- ◇ Find at least one thing, however small, for which you can express gratitude.

Appendix 2

Possible Interventions for Disturbing Behaviours in the Residential Aged Care Setting

<table>
<tr><th>Presenting Problems</th><th>Psycho-social Intervention</th></tr>
<tr><td>DEMENTIA

ALZHEIMER'S DISEASE

Common symptoms are:
• Cognitive symptoms: attention problems; memory (recent narrative recall); language-dysphasia; visuo-spatial dysfunction; praxis - apraxia; executive dysfunction – planning, organizing, abstraction, sequencing

• Affective disturbances: Depression, anxiety, agitation

• Psychotic delusion, hallucinations

• Sleep disturbance

• Apathetic syndrome

• Executive dysfunction syndrome: planning, organizing, abstraction, sequencing problems, personality change, disinhibition, verbal and motor perseveration</td><td>Potential strategies include:

• Integrating the Peaceful Mind and Open Heart approach and Mindfulness practices into all activities

• Reducing agitation and problem behaviours. The theoretical framework is based on:

• Behavioural model – ABC: Antecedent, Behaviour, Consequences

• Environmental vulnerability model:
Dementia results in increased vulnerability to the environment and lowers threshold of response to environmental or stressful stimulus</td></tr>
</table>

Presenting Problems	Psycho-social Intervention
DEMENTIA (continued) ALZHEIMER'S DISEASE • Eating problems: loss of interest in food, leads to poor nutrition May be related to: • Inflammatory process • Abnormal auto-immune modulation • Microvascular disease • Genetic aberrations (Adapted from Morris, P. 2015)	• Unmet needs model: Behaviours arise out of the difficulty that a person with dementia has in controlling their environment and in communicating their needs – problem behaviours can emerge as attempts to communicate those needs • Developing a plan that takes into account the unique individual characteristics and circumstances of the patient and the caring environment

Presenting Problems	Psycho-social Intervention
ANXIETY Common symptoms are: • Unrealistic fears • Excessive and uncontrollable worries • Behavioural agitation and irritability • Muscle tension • Sleep onset insomnia • Fatigue • Concentration problems • Heart palpitations • Shortness of breath and tightness in the chest May be related to: • Interpersonal symptoms • Change of environment • Grief • Pain • Isolation • Excess stimuli	Potential strategies include • Integrating the Peaceful Mind and Open Heart and Mindfulness approaches into all activities • Enhancing a sense of positive self-regard by reinforcing character strengths and positive achievements • Developing positive engagement in daily routines and social interactions • Developing positive health behaviours (e.g. healthy lifestyle choices) • Developing effective coping and problem solving skills • Exercise • Counselling / Cognitive Behaviour Therapy /Acceptance Committment Techniques • Reassurance with familiar objects • Reducing excessive stimuli • Increased involvement and collaboration with family and friends

Presenting Problems	Psycho-social Intervention
DEPRESSION Common symptoms are: • Sleep disturbance • Appetite or weight changes • Dysphoria (irritability or sadness) • Loss of interest in work, hobbies, etc. • Fatigue • Agitation or retardation • Diminished concentration • Low self-esteem or feelings of guilt • Suicidal thoughts May be related to: • Grief/bereavement • Change in environment • Past history of depression • Loss of familiar environment • Loss of roles • Change in self-image • Family history • Poor coping • Recent losses • Disease processes (Adapted from NSW Department of Health 2006)	Potential strategies include: • Integrating the Peaceful Mind and Open Heart and Mindfulness approaches into all activities • Enhancing a sense of positive self-regard by reinforcing character strengths and positive achievements • Developing positive engagement in daily routines and social interactions • Developing positive health behaviours (e.g. healthy lifestyle choices) • Developing effective coping and problem solving skills • Exercise • Counselling / Cognitive Behaviour Therapy /Acceptance Committment Techniques • Reassurance with familiar objects • Reducing excessive stimuli • Increased involvement and collaboration with family and friends • Pleasant events schedules

Presenting Problems	Psycho-social Intervention
AGGRESSION May be related to: • Pain • Frustration • Infection • Fear • Confusion • Psychosis • Excessive stimuli • Change of environment • Poor communication techniques • Loss of control • Drug reaction	Potential strategies include • Integrating the Peaceful Mind and Open Heart approach and Mindfulness practices into all activities • Distraction • Diversion • Music • Exercise • Avoidance of identified triggers • Appropriate levels of light • Reassurance with familiar objects • Family support • Noise and crowd reduction – peaceful environment • Assessment of family, social, psychological and occupational history • Socialisation

Presenting Problems	Psycho-social Intervention
AGITATION Is a multidimensional and complex phenomenon May be related to: • Anxiety • Pain • Discomfort • Constipation / Incontinence • Grief • Change of environment • Inappropriate medication regimes • Restraint (Adapted from NSW Department of Health 2006)	Potential strategies include: • Integrating the Peaceful Mind and Open Heart approach and Mindfulness practices into all activities • Modification of the environment • Provision of lounge chairs and sofas for companionship • Reassurance • Stimulation • Regular exercise • Signposting –cues • Asking the person if there is anything wrong • Distraction • Contact and closeness, where appropriate • Reducing crowding

Presenting Problems	Psycho-social Intervention
PSYCHOTIC SYMPTOMS Psychotic Symptoms include: • Delusions • Hallucinations • Paranoid ideation May be related to: • Misinterpretation of the environment • Drug toxicity/interactions • Visual or hearing impairment • Physical illness (Adapted from NSW Department of Health 2006)	Potential strategies include: • Integrating the Peaceful Mind and Open Heart approach and Mindfulness practices into all activities • Giving emotional support • Avoiding fatigue – encourage rest periods • Personalise environment / belongings • Having clear communication • Always keeping an open mind • Reducing stimulation and external stimuli e.g. TV, radio • Listening to their concerns and offer reassurance; however do not reinforce the delusions/paranoid ideations. This needs to be applied with respect for and sensitivity to the individuality of each situation • Investigating if there is any reality to what the person is saying

Presenting Problems	Psycho-social Intervention
SLEEP DISTURBANCES Include sleep-wake cycle problems May be related to: • Pain/joint stiffness • Poor mattress comfort • Nocturia • Noise (Adapted from NSW Department of Health 2006)	Potential strategies include: • Integrating the Peaceful Mind and Open Heart approach and Mindfulness practices into all activities • Investigate the night-time environment, including practices of night-staff disrupting residents' sleep • Creation of a sleeping environment • Night lights • Warm milk • Relaxation music • Caffeine restrictions • Limit daytime sleeping • Increase daytime exercise

Presenting Problems	Psycho-social Intervention
WANDERING May be related to: • Pacing associated with agitation • Restlessness associated with pain, anxiety frustration • Effect of medication • Stress • Boredom • Fear/loneliness • Isolation • Depression (Adapted from NSW Department of Health 2006)	Potential strategies include: • Asking the person what they are looking for or where they want to go • Identification • Use of alarms and monitors • Creating safe wandering opportunities • Walking programs • Exercise • Safe return programs • Diversions/distractions • Reminiscence therapy • Participating in household activities

<table>
<tr><th>Presenting Problems</th><th>Psycho-social Intervention</th></tr>
<tr><td>SUNDOWN SYNDROME (SUNDOWNING)

Sundowning is a state of agitation, confusion, anxiety and aggressiveness in late afternoon, in the evening or at night

May be related to:
• Inadequate exposure to amounts of light during the day
• Disturbance in circadian rhythm or changes in sleep-wake-cycles
• Sleep disorders (sleep disordered breathing and increased daytime napping)
• Less structured stimulation activity during the day which increases boredom, agitation and restlessness
• Medical and psychiatric condition

(Adapted from Khachiyants, et al, 2011)</td><td>Potential strategies include:
• Integrating the Peaceful Mind and Open Heart approach and Mindfulness practices into all activities
• Light therapy
• Music therapy
• Multisensory stimulation
• Reduction of noisy background, minimizing unnecessary noise
• Creating a comfortable and safe sleep environment</td></tr>
</table>

Activities associated with potential behavioural and psychological symptoms of dementia (BPSD)	Behaviour Management Intervention
• Bathing	Make a safe bathroom. Be prepared, don't rush. Ensure room and water temperature are comfortable. Wash hair last. A recent study found that the benefits of person-centered bathing and towel bath were shown to be decreasing agitation and discomfort expressed by the person being cared for.
• Dressing	Limit choices. Prepare clothing. Give specific cues. Provide larger clothing and soft stretchy fabrics. Provide duplicate outfits and comfortable shoes with Velcro. Give positive reinforcement.
• Eating	Maintain a regular mealtime schedule. Avoid distraction at mealtimes. Check the food temperature. Honour preferences when possible, and offer finger foods.
• Wandering	Provide adequate daily physical activity. Create a safe environment and safe wandering paths. Remove reminders of leaving (coats, umbrella). Have alarms or bells at exit doors.
• Incontinence (Adapted from Sloane et al 2004)	Scheduled voiding. Be attentive to nonverbal cues (such as pacing). Simplify clothing and clear obstacles. Put signs (including pictures) at the bathroom door. Give positive reinforcement.

References and Readings

Aked, J., Marks, N., et al. (2008). Five Ways to Wellbeing: The evidence. A report presented to the Foresight Project on *Communicating the Evidence Base for Improving People's Wellbeing*.

Aldwin, C.M., Park, C.L., & Spiro III, A. (2007). *Handbook of Health, Psychology and Aging.*

Alzheimer's Disease International. *World Alzheimer Report 2009: The Global Prevalence of Dementia.*

Baer, R.A., et al. (2006). Using Self-report Assessment Methods to Explore Facets of Mindfulness. In *Assessment, 2006, 13 (1).*

Barrick, A.L., Rader, J., et al. (2008). *Bathing Without a Battle: Person-Directed Care of Individuals with Dementia.*

Berger, R. (2003). *An Ethic of Excellence: Building a Culture of Craftsmanship with Students.*

Bernhard, T. (2013). How *to Wake Up: A Buddhist Inspired Guide to Navigating Joy and Sorrow.*

Biglan, A., et al. (2012). The Critical Role of Nurturing Environments for Promoting Human Wellbeing. In *American Psychologist, 2012, 67 (4).*

Bishop, S., Lau, M., Carlson, L., et al. (2004). Mindfulness: A Proposed Operational Definition. In *Clinical Psychology Science & Practice, 2004, 11 (3).*

Brodaty, H., Draper, B.M., & Low, L.F. (2003). Behavioral and Psychological Symptoms of Dementia: a seven-tiered model of service delivery. In *Medical Journal of Australia, 2003, 178 (5).*

Brownie, S., & Nancarrow, S. (2013). Effects of person-centered care on residents and staff in aged-care facilities: A systematic review. In *Journal of Clinical Interventions in Aging, 2013, 8.*

Browning, C., Gridley, H., Helmes, E., et al. (2000). *Psychology and Aging.* A Position Paper prepared for the Australian Psychological Society, May 2000.

Buhler, C. (1961). Meaningful living in the mature years. In Kleemeier, R.W. *Aging and Leisure: A Research perspective into the Meaningful Use of Time, 1961.*

Burns, K., Jayasintha, R., & Brodaty, H. (2012). Behavioral Management – A Guide to Good Practice : Managing Behavioral and Psychological Symptoms of Dementia (BPSD). In *Dementia Collaborative Research Centre – Assessment and Better Care.*

Cabeza, R., et al. (2002). Aging gracefully: Compensatory brain activity in high-performing older Adults. In *NeuroImage, 2002, 17.*

Cameron, J.I., & Gignac, M.A.M. (2008). Timing It Right: A conceptual framework for addressing the support needs of family caregivers to stroke survivors from the hospital to the home. In *Patient Education Counselling, 2008, 70 (3).*

Carstensen, L. (2007). Growing Old or Living Long: Take Your Pick. In *Science and Technology, 2007, 23 (2).*

Cassidy, J., & Shaver, P.R. (2008). *Handbook of Attachment: Theory, Research and Clinical Applications.*

Childre, D., & McCraty, R. (2001). Psychophysiological Correlates of Spiritual Experience. In *Association of Applied Psychophysiology and Biofeedback (AAPB) & Biofeedback Magazine, 2001, 29 (4).*

Childre, D., & Howard, M. (2011). *The Heartmath Solution.*

Condon, P., Desbordes, G., et al. (2013). Meditation Increases Compassionate Responses to Suffering. In *Psychological Science, August 2013, 24.*

Coyle, D. (2009). *The Talent Code: Greatness Isn't Born. It's Grown. Here's How.*

Crick, F. (1979). Thinking About the Brain. In *The Brain: A Scientific American Book.*

Cullen, M. (2011). Mindfulness-Based Interventions: An Emerging Phenomenon. In *Mindfulness, September 2011, 2 (3).*

Cummins, R., & Nistico, H. (2002). Maintaining Life Satisfaction: The Role of Positive Cognitive Bias. In *Journal of Happiness Studies, 2002, 3 (1).*

Danner, D.D., Snowdon, D.A., & Friesen, W.V. (2001). Positive Emotions in Early Life and Longevity: Findings from the Nun study. In *Journal of Personality and Social Psychology, 2001, 80 (5).*

Davidson, R. (2008). Buddha's Brain: Neuroplasticity and Meditation. In *Signal Processing Magazine, 2008, 25(1).*

Davidson, R., & Begley, S. (2012). *The Emotional Life of your Brain: How its Unique Patterns Affect the Way You Think, Feel and Live and How You Can Change Them.*

DeSteno, D., & Condon, P. (2013). Can meditation make you a more compassionate person? In *Association for Psychological Science, April 2013.*

Dementia in Australia (2012). Report prepared by: Vanden Heuvel, A., Hudson, C., & Cargill, J. Australia Institute of Health and Welfare.

Dennett, D.C. (1992). The Self as a Centre of Narrative Gravity. In Kessel, F., Cole, P.M., and Johnson, D. *Self and Consciousness: Multiple Perspectives, 1992.*

Depression in Older Age: A Scoping Study (2009). Final Report prepared by Haralambous, B., Lin, X., et al. Natural Aging Research Institute.

Diefenbach, G.J., & Goethe, J. (2006). Clinical Interventions for Late-life Anxious Depression. In *Journal of Clinical Intervention in Aging, 2006, 1 (1).*

Doidge, N. (2007). *The Brain that Changes Itself: Stories of Personal Triumph from the Frontiers of Brain Science.*

Doidge, N. (2015). *The Brain's Way of Healing: Remarkable Discoveries and Recoveries from the Frontiers of Neuroplasticity.*

Draper, B. (2011). *Understanding Alzheimer's & other Dementias.*

Dresler, M., Wehrie, R., Spoormaker,V.I., et al. (2012). The Seat of Meta-Consciousness in the Brain. In *Max-Planck Institute of Psychiatry, Cognitive Science, July 2012.*

Egan, N. (2014). Secret to aged care happiness. In *Australian Ageing Agenda, August 2014.*

Emoto, M. (2004). *The Hidden Messages in Water.*

Feeney, B. C., & Collins, N.L. (2014). A New Look at Social Support: A Theoretical Perspective on Thriving through Relationships. In *Personality and Social Psychology Review, 2014.*

Frankl, V. (1964). *Man's Search for Meaning: An Introduction to Logotherapy.*

Gawande, A. (2014). *Being Mortal: Medicine and What Matters in the End.*

Gerdner, L.A. (2005). Use of individualized music by trained staff and family: Translating research into practice. In *Journal of Gerontological Nursing, 2005, (6).*

Gerzon, R. (1997). *Finding Serenity in the Age of Anxiety.*

Glisky, E.L. (2007). Changes in Cognitive Function in Human Aging. In Riddle, D.R. *Brain Aging: Models, Methods, and Mechanisms.*

Goleman, D. (1995). *Emotional Intelligence: Why it can matter more than IQ.*

Graham, L. (2008). The Neuroscience of Attachment. First presented as a *Clinical Conversation at the Community Institute for Psychotherapy.*

Graham, L. (2013). *Bouncing Back. Rewiring your Brain for Maximum Resilience and Well-being.*

Gross, J.J. (2014). *Handbook of Emotion Regulation.*

Guidelines for Working with People with Challenging Behaviors in Residential Aged Care Facilities. NSW Department of Health, 2006.

Gurdjieff, G.J. (1999). *Life is Real only Then, When 'I am'.*

Hanson, R., & Mencius, R. (2009). *Buddha's Brain. The Practical Neuroscience of Happiness, Love and Wisdom.*

Harris, R. (2007). *The Happiness Trap. Stop Struggling, Start Living.*

Hayes, S.C., & Strosahl, K. (2004). *A Practical Guide to Acceptance and Commitment Therapy.*

Hersch, E.C., & Falzgraf, S. (2007). Management of the behavioral and psychological symptoms of dementia. In *Journal of Clinical Interventions in Aging, 2007, 2 (4).*

Inmordino-Yang, M.H., & Damasio, A. (2007). We Feel, Therefore We Learn. The Relevance of Affective and Social Neuroscience to Education. In *Mind, Brain and Education, 1, (1).*

Immordino-Yang, M.H., et al. (2009). Neural correlates of admiration and compassion. In *Proceedings of the National Academy of Sciences of USA, 106 (19).*

Jacoby, R., et al. (2008). *Oxford Textbook of Old Age Psychiatry.*

Jeffers, S. (2007). *Feel the Fear and do it Anyway.*

Kabat-Zinn, J. (1990). *Full Catastrophe Living: Using the Wisdom of your Body and Mind to face Stress, Pain and Illness.*

Kabat-Zinn, J. (1994). *Wherever you go, there you are. Mindfulness Meditation in Everyday Life.*

Khachiyants, N., et al. (2011). Sundown Syndrome in Persons with Dementia: An update. In *Psychiatry Investigation, 2011, 8 (4).*

Kinsella, G., et al. (2010). Cognitive Interventions in early Alzheimer's Disease and mild Cognitive Impairment. In *InPsych, 2010, 32 (5).*

Kornfield, J. (2008). *The Wise Heart: Buddhist Psychology for the West.*

Kryla-Lighthall, N., & Maher, M. (2009). The Role of Cognitive Control in Older Adults' Emotional Wellbeing. In Bengtson, V., Gans, D., Putney, N., & Silverstein, M. *Handbook of Theories of Aging.*

Kunzmann, U., Little, T., & Smith, J. (2002). Perceiving Control: A Double-edged Sword in Old Age. In *Journal of Gerontology. Series B: Psychological Sciences and Social Sciences, 2002, 57B (6).*

Lacey, B., & Lacey, J. (1978). Two-way Communication between the Heart and the Brain: Significance of time within the Cardiac Cycle. In *American Psychologist, 1978, 33 (2).*

Lee, H., & Adams, T. (2011). *Creative Approaches in Dementia Care.*

Lomas, T., et al. (2016). Mindful Living in Older Age: A Pilot Study of a Brief, Community-based Positive Aging Intervention. In *Mindfulness, 2016, 7 (3).*

Lopez Ulloa, B.F., Moller, V., & Sousa-Poza, A. (2013). *How does Subjective Well-being Evolve with Age? A Literature Review.*

Lykken, D. (2000). *Happiness: The Nature and Nurture of Joy and Contentment.*

Lyubomirsky, S. (2008). *The How of Happiness: A New Approach to Getting the Life You Want.*

Machado de Lima, A.M., Salmazo da Silva, H., & Galhardoni, R. (2008). Successful aging:Paths for a construct and new frontiers. In *Interface (Botucatu), 2008, 12 (27).*

Mackenzie, E.R., & Rakel, B. (2006). *Complementary and Alternative Medicine for Older Adults.*

Maher, M. (2016). The Affective Neuroscience of Aging. In *Annual Review of Psychology, 2016, 67.*

Manepalli, J., et al. (2009). Psychosocial – Environmental Treatments for Alzheimer's Disease. In *Primary Psychiatry, 2009, 16 (6).*

Mantamadiotis, T. (2012). *When Things Go Wrong - Diseases and Disorders of the Human Brain.*

McCabe, M.P., et al. (2013). A study protocol to investigate the management of depression and challenging behaviors associated with dementia in aged care settings. In *BioMed Central (BMC) Geriatrics, 2013, 13 (95).*

McCraty, R., Atkinson, M., & Tomasino, D. (2001). *Science of the Heart. Exploring the Role of the Heart in Human Performance.* An overview of research conducted by The Institute of HeartMath.

McCraty, R. (2002). Heart Rhythm Coherence: An Emerging Area of Biofeedback. In *Association of Applied Psychophysiology and Biofeedback (AAPB) and Biofeedback magazine, 2002, 30 (1).*

McCraty, R., & Zayas, M.A. (2014). Cardiac Coherence, Self-regulation, Autonomic Stability, and Psychosocial Wellbeing. In *Frontiers in Psychology, 2014, 5.*

McGrath, H., & Noble, T. (2003). *Bounce Back: A Classroom Resiliency Program.*

McGrath, H., & Noble, T. (2011). *Bounce Back: A Wellbeing & Resilience Program.*

McGrath, H., & Noble, T. (2012). Well-being and resilience in young people and the role of positive relationships. In Roffey, S. *Positive Relationships: Evidence-based Practice Across the World.*

Minsky, M. (2006). *The Emotion Machine: Commonsense Thinking, Artificial Intelligence, and the Future of the Human Mind.*

Moorjani, A. (2012). *Dying to be Me: My Journey from Cancer, to Near Death, to True Healing.*

Morris, P. (2015). New Developments in Alzheimer's Disease. In *Springfield Advances in Alzheimer's Treatment Conference, Athens, 2016.*

Newberg, A., & D'Aquili, E. (2002). *Why God won't go away: Brain Science and the Biology of Belief.*

Norcross, J.C. (2002). *Psychotherapy Relationships That Work: Therapist Contributions and Responsiveness to Patients.*

Nouwen, H. (2009). *The Way of the Heart: The Spirituality of the Desert Fathers and Mothers.*

O'Donohue, J. (2012). *An Abundance of Blessings: 52 Meditations to Illuminate Your Life.*

Orage, A.R. (1976). *Psychological Exercises and Essays.*

Palmo, Tenzin. (2002). *Reflections on a Mountain Lake: Teaching on Practical Buddhism.*

Pargament, K. (1997). *The Psychology of Religion: Theory, research, practice.*

Porges, S.W. (2011). *The Polyvagal theory: Neurophysiological Foundations of Emotions, Attachment, Communication, Self-regulation.*

Ram Dass (1971). *Be Here Now.*

Ram Dass (2000). *Still Here. Embracing Aging, Changing, and Dying.*

Ramana Maharshi (1972). *The Spiritual Teaching of Ramana Maharshi.*

Rahhal, T.A., May, C.P., & Hasher, L. (2002). Truth and Character: Sources that Older Adults can Remember. In *Psychological Science, March 2002, 13 (2).*

Raz, N., & Rodrigue, K.M. (2006). Differential Aging of the Brain: Patterns, cognitive correlates and modifiers. In *Neuroscience and Biobehavioral Reviews, 2006, 30 (6).*

Reuter-Lorenz, P.A., & Park, D.C. (2010). Human Neuroscience and the Aging Mind: A New look at Old Problems. In *The Journal of Gerontology. Series B: Psychological Sciences of Social Sciences 2010, 65B (4).*

Ricard, M. (2013). *Altruism. The Power of Compassion to Change Yourself and the World.*

Richmond, L. (2012). *Aging as a Spiritual Practice. A Contemplative Guide to Growing Older and Wiser.*

Richo, D. (2002). *How to Be an Adult in Relationships: The Five Keys to Mindful Loving.*

Rock, D., Siegel, D., Poelmans, S., & Payne, J. (2011). The Healthy Mind Platter. In *NeuroLeadership Journal, 4, 40 – 62.*

Rowe, J., & Kahn, R. (1999). *Successful Aging*.

Scheibe, S., & Carstensen, L.L. (2010). Emotional Aging: Recent Findings and Future Trends. In *Journal of Gerontology: Psychological Sciences, 2010, 65B 135 - 144.*

Scommegna, P. (2016). Today's Research on Aging: Family Caregiving. In *Population Reference Bureau, February, 2016.*

Seeher, K., Withall, A., & Brodaty, H. (2011). The Dementia Research Mapping Project: The 2010 Update: Final report. In *Dementia Collaborative Research Centre, Assessment and Better Care, Sydney, April 2011*.

Seligman, M., Reivich, K., Jaycox, L., & Gillham, J. (1995). *The Optimistic Child.*

Seligman, M. (2002). *Authentic Happiness: Using the New Positive Psychology to Realize Your Potential for Lasting Fulfillment.*

Seligman, M., & Peterson, C. (2004). *Character Strengths and Virtues: A Handbook and Classification.*

Seligman, M. (2011). *Flourish: A Visionary New Understanding of Happiness and Well-being.*

Sheldon, K.M., & Lyubomirsky, S. (2006). How to increase and sustain positive emotion:The effects of expressing gratitude and visualizing best possible selves. In *The Journal Of Positive Psychology, April 2006, 1 (2).*

Siegel, B. (1998). *Peace, Love and Healing. Bodymind Communication & the Path to Self-Healing: An exploration.*

Siegel, D. (2007). *The Mindful Brain. Reflection and Attunement in the Cultivation of Well-Being.*

Siegel, D. (2010). *The Mindful Therapist: A Clinician's Guide to Mindsight and Neural Integration.*

Siegel, D. (2010). *Mindsight. The New Science of Personal Transformation.*

Siegel, D., & Bryson, T. (2011). *The Whole Brain Child: 12 Revolutionary Strategies to Nurture Your Child's developing Mind.*

Siegel, D., Siegel, M., & Parker, S. (2012). *Internal Education and the Roots of Resilience.*

Siegel, D. (2012). *The Developing Mind. How Relationships and the Brain Interact to Shape Who we Are.*

Sloane, P.D., Hoeffer, B., Mitchell, C.M., et al. (2004). Effect of person-centered showering and the towel bath on bathing- associated aggression, agitation, and discomfort in nursing home residents with dementia: a randomized, controlled trial. In *Journal of the American Geriatrics Society, 2004, 52 (11).*

Smalley, S., & Winston, D. (2010). *Fully Present: The Science, Art and Practice of Mindfulness.*

Steptoe, A., Deaton, A., & Stone, A.A. (2015). Subjective Wellbeing, Health and Ageing. In the *Lancet, Feb. 14, 2015.*

Sung, H.C., Chang, A. M., & Abbey, J. (2010). A preferred music listening intervention to reduce anxiety in older adults with dementia in nursing homes. In *Clinical Nursing, 2010, 19.*

Talbot, M. (1991). *The Holographic Universe.*

Thich Nhat Hanh (1987). *Being Peace.*

Thich Nhat Hanh (1992). *Touching Peace: Practicing the Art of Mindful Living.*

Thomas, L. (1974). *The Lives of a Cell: Notes of a Biology Watcher.*

Thomas, W. (1994). *The Eden Alternative: Nature, Hope and Nursing Homes.*

Tolle, E. (1997). *The Power of Now.*

Ungar, M. (2014). *Report of the 2014 Thinker in Residence:Resilience.* Commissioner for Children and Young People Western Australia.

Valentine, M. (2016). *Living Zen Spirit.*

Vivekananda (1993). *Living at the Source: Yoga Teachings of Vivekananda.*

Waring, A. (2012). *The Heart of Care: Dignity in Action: A Guide to Person-centred Compassionate Elder Care.*

Warneken, F., & Tomasello, M. (2009). The roots of human altruism. In *British Journal of Psychology, 100, 455-471.*

Watts, A. (1940). The Meaning of Happiness: The Quest for Freedom of the Spirit. In *Modern Psychology & the Wisdom of the East.*

Wells, Y., Bhar, S., Kinsella, G., et al. (2014). What works to promote emotional wellbeing in older people. A guide for aged care staff working in community or residential care settings. In *Beyondblue Publication (2014).*

Wetherill, L., et al. (2011). Acceptance and Commitment Therapy for Generalized Adults: A preliminary report. In *Behaviour Therapy, 42, 127 – 134.*

Williamson, M. (1992). *A Return to Love. Reflections on the Principles of A Course in Miracles.*

Wong, P.T.P. (2010). *Spirituality and Aging*.

Zahavi, D. (2011). The Experiential Self: Objections and Clarifications. In Siderits, M., Thompson, E., & Zahavi, D. *Self, No Self? Perspectives from Analytical, Phenomenological, and Indian Traditions (2010)*

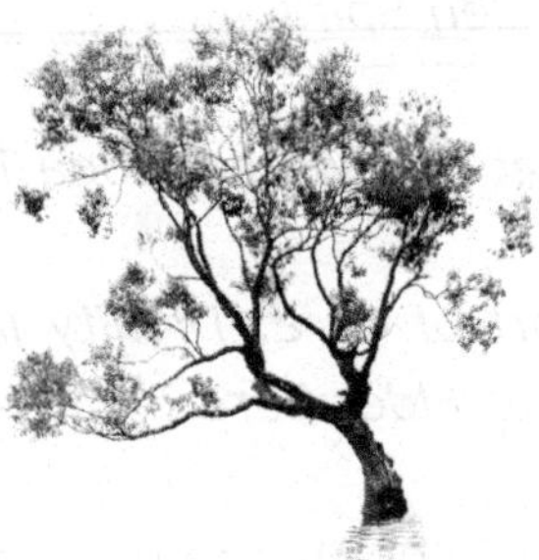

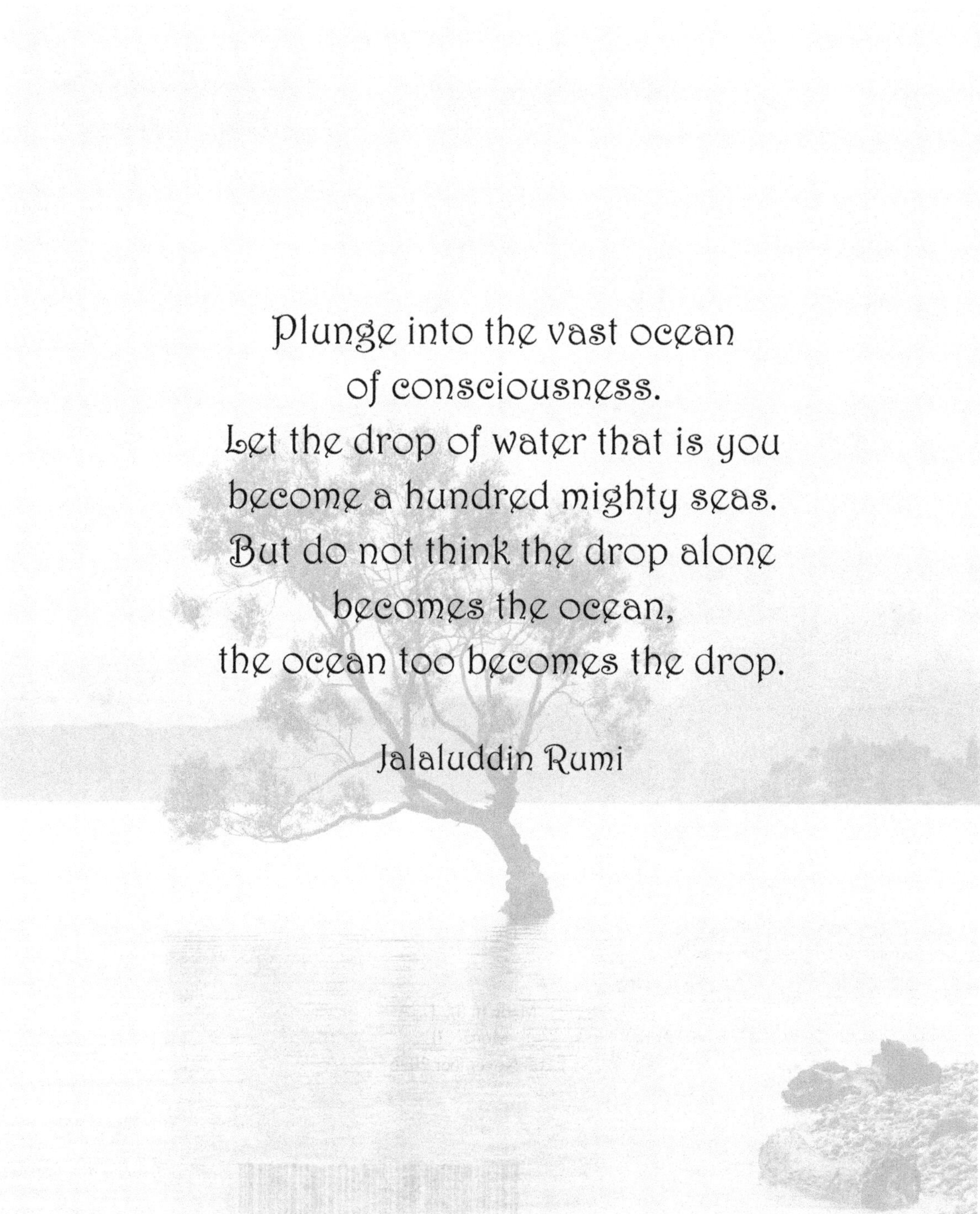

Plunge into the vast ocean
of consciousness.
Let the drop of water that is you
become a hundred mighty seas.
But do not think the drop alone
becomes the ocean,
the ocean too becomes the drop.

Jalaluddin Rumi

Made in the USA
Monee, IL
08 November 2026

67944854R00181